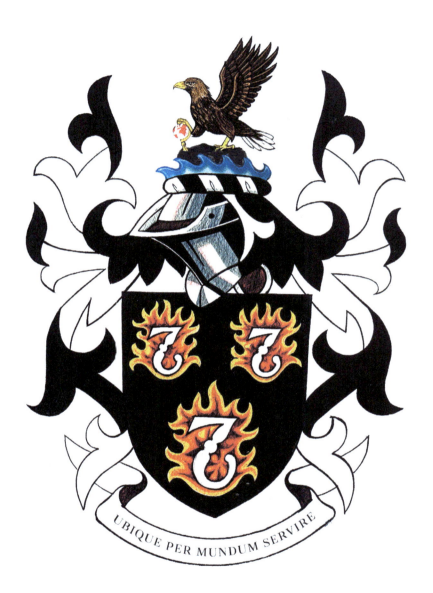

The arms and crest of
Professor Anthony Roberts OBE OStJ

SCHOLARSHIP BOY TO ENGINEER, PLASTIC SURGEON AND SPORTSMAN

PROFESSOR ANTHONY ROBERTS OBE FRCS

Copyright © 2022 Professor Anthony Roberts OBE FRCS

The moral right of the author has been asserted.

Apart from any fair dealing for the purposes of research or private study, or criticism or review, as permitted under the Copyright, Designs and Patents Act 1988, this publication may only be reproduced, stored or transmitted, in any form or by any means, with the prior permission in writing of the publishers, or in the case of reprographic reproduction in accordance with the terms of licences issued by the Copyright Licensing Agency. Enquiries concerning reproduction outside those terms should be sent to the publishers.

Matador
Unit E2 Airfield Business Park
Harrison Road, Market Harborough
Leics LE16 7UL
Tel: 0116 279 2299
Email: books@troubador.co.uk
Web: www.troubador.co.uk/matador
Twitter: @matadorbooks

ISBN 978 1 80313 525 0

British Library Cataloguing in Publication Data.
A catalogue record for this book is available from the British Library.

Printed and bound by CPI Group (UK) Ltd, Croydon, CR0 4YY
Typeset in 11pt Minion Pro by Troubador Publishing Ltd, Leicester, UK

Matador is an imprint of Troubador Publishing Ltd

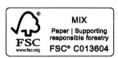

I am dedicating this book to my late mother, Ivy Roberts

Without her not only would I not be here, but without her dedication during my early and difficult years I would certainly not be where I am today.

All profits from the sale of this book will be given to
'Restore – Burn and Wound Research'
A medical research charity that I created some thirty years ago with the aims of reducing scarring from burns or from any other cause.

The next part of my professional life is being published within a few months and is entitled
Plastic Surgery in Wars, Disasters and Civilian Life.

CONTENTS

Foreword		ix
Introduction		xi
PART 1	**ENGINEERING**	**1**
1	University of Leeds	3
2	University of Cambridge – Research	14
3	The Chemical Engineer	25
PART 2	**MEDICINE AND PLASTIC SURGERY**	**37**
4	University of Cambridge – Undergraduate	39
5	University of Zambia	49
6	University of Oxford	63
7	University of the Witswatersrand	80
8	University of Michigan	94
9	House Officer	101
10	Southern Africa	112
11	Senior House Officer and Registrar	126
12	Microsurgery in Australia	179
13	Consultant at last	182
PART 3	**SPORT**	**185**
Introduction		187
14	Soccer and Rugby	189
15	Cricket	193

16	Badminton, Squash and Tennis	199
17	Swimming, SCUBA Diving, Canoeing and Rowing	208
18	Athletics	215
19	Ice Hockey and Field Hockey	218
20	Skiing	224
21	Sailing	234
22	Training and other sports	257
PART 4	**RELIGION, POLITICS AND RACE**	**261** |//
Summary		274
Afterthoughts		275
References		279
Index		281

FOREWORD

I returned from New York in 1967 and was delighted to be a member of the Graduates' Parlour at St Catharine's College, Cambridge. An early meeting was with this sophisticated academic who was taking an undergraduate course, a medic. Anthony was embarking on a new career. He was already an established lecturer in engineering, but he clearly had a higher calling.

This was an active community with learning on many dimensions. Our academic progress was important but so were other things. Anthony had influence. He taught me to sail a dinghy. This small beginning spurred me on to a Fastnet Race and two China Sea Races. Always a sportsman, Anthony played ice hockey for the University. The Cam was a major influence, we both rowed. We took to skiing. Later with children and grandchildren. One of the great joys of life.

But Anthony's strongest influence was the world experience he added to all our vigorous discussions. He had assets, which the rest of the community did not have. He accumulated books more rapidly than anyone I know. He had been places and done things that we could only dream about. But degrees were achieved, and work followed, with much travel for us all.

I was delighted to introduce Vivian to Anthony when her medical houseman perambulations took her to Oxford, and what a good introduction that was. They married!

Watching from afar, Anthony's specialism in surgery, and in trauma surgery, seemed a natural progression for one who combines a worldwide view with detailed competencies in science, both in medicine and in engineering. Anthony is a practical fixer. Clearly his appetite for fixing things as an engineer moved on to fixing people as a doctor and then to fixing their wounds as a trauma surgeon and on to some "fixing" of medical research with his charity and fixing other countries health delivery with his international teaching and work.

He was always a very disciplined workaholic. And his memoirs shows that has not faded.

This autobiography is a treasure house of memories, more detailed than I could ever imagine. Memories of people and events are interleaved with descriptions of university structures and university life. Clearly Anthony was hyperactive, and that continues to this day. His was involved in a superb range of academic activities, studying and teaching at the same time, and a superb range of sporting activities at a very high level.

We have never discussed fluidized bed technology. It is not a subject of everyday conversation. But it is an important aspect of my own work in decarbonisation of industrial processes. Anthony is unfairly downbeat about the failure of his research project; deep learning comes as much from the projects that don't work as those which do. A discussion for another day.

There are career development lessons here for the aspiring sixth former through to the budding consultant surgeon. Networking is a valuable life skill, demonstrated by Anthony at a high level. I am sure you will learn from this excursion into a life of highly sophisticated medicine, and we will all be better off as a result.

Dr Brian Sweeney

INTRODUCTION

This book is about my education, my training and my work as an engineer, and then my qualification as a doctor and my training as a surgeon until I was appointed as a consultant plastic and hand surgeon at Stoke Mandeville Hospital in 1985. It includes sport which was an important part of that period of my life. I received university colours in badminton, half-blues at Cambridge and Oxford and British Universities colours for ice-hockey, and university and British Universities colours in sailing as well as competing in the Olympic trials.

I have published my work as a plastic surgeon in Britain and around the world in the second volume of my memoirs *Plastic Surgery in Wars, Disasters and Civilian Life*, and next intend to publish my family life, my schooling and my hobbies. This latter will I am sure be of more interest to my family members. If I live long enough a volume on my travels within Great Britain and to 107 countries, and the biological work that I have done both in Great Britain and overseas will follow.

A few sentences about myself. I was born in Woodford Wells in Essex in 1938 as the only child of Kenneth Arthur Norman Roberts and Ivy Beatrice Maude Roberts (née Leggatt) after five years of their marriage. My father was a timber salesman and my mother a shorthand typist. At the beginning of the Second World War my father joined the Royal Air Force Volunteer Reserve as an administrative officer. We lived in Scotland and at various bases in England as he was posted around the country. As the war was finishing my parents separated and were subsequently divorced. At that time I had caught TB and was spending time in various hospitals or living with my mother in the houses of two of her brothers and their families. By daily injections of streptomycin for three months I was eventually cured of TB. I still remember the injections! What I do not remember is any schooling in the hospitals and my mother, although uneducated, must have taught me the three Rs, Reading, Riting and Rithmetic. After the war we returned to the two-bedroomed bungalow which mother had acquired as part of the divorce settlement, but she still needed to pay off the remainder of the mortgage. To do this she had to take a variety of paying guests who occupied half the bungalow. I had the boxroom which measured 8' by 5' as my bedroom and later study.

When I was nearly eight I started at Woodford Green Primary School and three years later I very fortuitously won a scholarship to Bancroft's School, a local public school. My mother's finances were such that the scholarship even paid for my school uniform. From there I won another scholarship to read engineering at the University of Leeds, and that is the start of this book.

My change to medicine came ten years later, again on a further scholarship. Chapters 4 to 8 describe my qualification as a doctor, and chapters 9 to 13 my training as a surgeon and then as a plastic surgeon. Having started ten years behind my colleagues and competitors for posts I spent those thirteen years trying to catch up by filling every possible gap doing locum appointments between the main training posts. This gave me a more extensive experience than most young surgeons. I have worked out that I worked for, and was taught by ten general surgeons, seven orthopaedic or accident surgeons and eighteen plastic surgeons. In retrospect learning something, nearly always but not always good, from each one has been incredibly useful in my career. And I did catch up five years on all but one of my colleagues.

The third part of this book is about sport. Sport was an extremely important part of my life at school, at universities and to a lesser degree for the rest of my life. Much of my non working time and my friends have come about through sport. It is interesting that the part of one's character that makes one a good successful sportsman I believe is the same as that required to become a good surgeon.

The final short section are my views on life – on religion, politics and race. All of these have been important and their input into my life has changed, and still continues to change as my life nears its end.

Part One

Engineering

ONE

UNIVERSITY OF LEEDS

At the beginning of my last year at school I had had a discussion with an Old Bancroftian about possible future careers after the A-level examinations had finished. The person who interviewed me was Mr Ned Warner. I had previously decided that my career was to be as a chemist. We had a discussion about the chances of me getting brilliant results in my A-level examinations, and being quite honest I said this was unlikely. Mr Warner suggested that unless I was guaranteed to get a first class degree, I should consider chemical engineering. It was many years later that I discovered that Mr Warner was in fact a very successful chemical engineer, later to be knighted for his services to the industry, and also elected a Fellow of the Royal Society. Perhaps he was a little biased.

Not long after my interview with Mr Warner my mother noticed in a paper that there was an industrial scholarship advertised by the British Coke Research Association (BCRA) which would pay considerably more money than the normal university scholarships which were available from the Essex County Council. Being honest both then and now, I knew nothing about the coking industry, and very little indeed about the coal industry in Britain. However the possibility of a better grant made me apply. My application was accepted, and I went up for a long interview in London at the National Coal Board. I have very little memories of this interview but somehow I must have impressed them because they offered me a scholarship. I then had the decision to make as to which universities I wished to apply. Imperial College London was certainly the best known department of chemical engineering in Britain, but I also applied to other universities including Manchester and Leeds.

Some months later I took my four A-levels, but before knowing the results of the exams I was on a boat to Arctic Lapland with the British Schools Exploring Society.

In those days there were no simple telephone or radio connections, except for absolute emergencies, between home and those of us who were in the field some hundreds of miles north of the Arctic Circle. It was not therefore until I was on my way home that I received the news I had passed three of the four A-levels, with a close miss in the fourth. I also discovered, and not to my surprise at all, that Imperial College had not offered me a place, but that Leeds University had. It turned out that the British Coke Research Association scholarship preferred me to do the course in gas engineering at Leeds together with two other scholars who had been appointed at the same time. Tragically one of these died from Hodgkin's lymphoma which was then incurable during the second year long vacation

As well as the four years of funding for my university, the Association also paid for a three day conference each year where one met people within the industry, people from the trade unions, and other relevant academics. Before starting at Leeds I therefore went to the conference at Tring in Hertfordshire, and was allocated a mentor with whom I would have some contact over the next four years. He was the coke oven manager in Rotherham at that time.

At the end of the conference he very kindly drove me to Leeds. At that time all undergraduates, even those over 21 without parent's permission lived at home or stayed either in a Hall of Residence or were in allocated diggings. I had not applied to a Hall because of my travels overseas, and was therefore allocated digs in Bramley. Bramley was, and is, a small township about 4 to 5 miles north-west of the city centre on the Bradford road. As we drove into Bramley, I very nearly changed my mind about going to university at all. It was a very dirty small miserable little town where the houses were often in rows and mostly with outside loos. However the digs that I had been allocated were No. 31 Town Street, and by very lucky chance this was the only nice and elegant house in the whole street. It was of late Georgian or possibly early Victorian construction standing in some 2 to 3 acres of grounds. I knocked on the door to be met by my new landlady, Mrs Fishburn. She was an enormously cheerful and very pleasant lady with a classical Yorkshire accent and also with

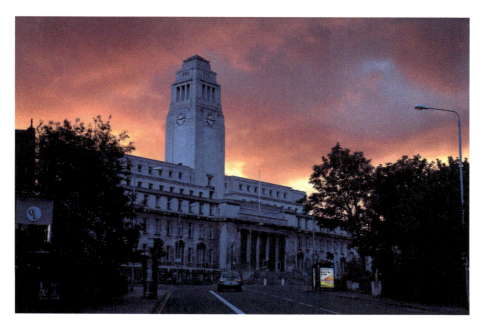

1.1 The Parkinson Building of the University of Leeds

the slightly large figure of a typical well off Yorkshire lady. Her husband Jack had a business in the grounds of the house making and repairing cars, lorries and coaches.

The whole situation therefore became considerably brighter. I then met the other two new undergraduates who had also being allocated that year to the house where we would join four others who had been there the previous year.

The University of Leeds was a typical redbrick university. In fact very little of it was redbrick but made of very elegant Portland stone. (Photo 1.1). It had been founded in 1904 and became independent in 1930. In 1957 when I joined it there were some 3500 students of whom approximately one third were engineers, one quarter scientists and the rest spread between a variety of subjects. The engineering school was in two separate parts. The normal engineering subjects of civil, mechanical and electrical were just north of the main university buildings, and in a new building known as the Houldsworth School of Applied Science even further north of that were the departments of chemical engineering, gas engineering, fuel science, metallurgy and ceramics. There were some 50 chemical engineering students in each academic year, 15 gas engineering, 30 to 40 fuel science undergraduates and about 10 undergraduates studying ceramics. The whole of the Houldsworth School was in some confusion at the time, with no appointed Professor. However several of the lecturers had been there for several years. Within gas engineering there was Dr Gartside in charge, and Mr McRae and Dr Roberts as the second level of lecturer. I will enlarge on these later.

And so term started. As is now absolutely normal, but still occurred even in 1957 at Leeds, there were an introductory three days for the new students. This consisted of several lectures about the University, about how to study, and other general lectures from our departments about what we had been recruited to study. It was also an opportunity for the various sports and other clubs within the University to recruit people with a variety of stands where one could find out about the clubs, and the cost of each. The three that I joined straightaway were the Sailing Club at a cost of five shillings a year (25p), the Natural History Society, and the Rover Scouts. I looked at the possibility of other clubs, and in particular various sports clubs but at that stage decided not to join any of them as I was not sure what my finances would bear. I also still had some effects from the broken wrist of that spring. I will go into details about the sailing club in chapter 21. The Scouts will be in my next book. The Natural History Society, although I was a member, I had in fact very little to do with it during my first year, and did not renew my subscription as I was already more committed to other interests.

Looking back over my years in Leeds, where one's digs and flatmates were an incredibly important part of one's social life, I was extremely lucky with my allocated digs in those first two years, and with the people who were already there, and those who came in with me. The seven of us were allocated to four rooms, with Neil Stevenson, very much the elder statesman of us because of his previous career, having the single room, and the rest of us shared. Again I was lucky to be sharing with Roger Dunn – apart from his unbelievably smelly feet to which changing his socks regularly made no difference – who was also a chemical engineering student the year above me. Of the seven of us three of us were in the Houldsworth School of Applied Science, Howard Toon was a mechanical engineer, Neil Stevenson was a pharmacologist, Don Mallick a geologist and David Stevenson a chemist. One might say, and I know many people would, that with scientists and engineers only there was very little educated discussion in the digs. This was to some extent true, but sport was very much part of our lives. Of the seven of us, five of us obtained University colours. Roger Dunn had been a schoolboy soccer international, and Don

Mallick had been fourth in the national junior shot putt championships and had had an amazing school athletic background. There was also a strong Christian element within the group. Both Roger Dunn and Neil Stevenson were strict Methodists, which had a great disadvantage for a trip to the pub, three of us were quite serious members of the Church of England and the other two considered religion was of less importance.

As I said earlier the house was large and elegant. Next door to the house was the Bramley rugby league football ground, and through our bathroom window one could see three quarters of the field. Next door again to that was a public house, the Barley Mow. We would go there on occasions, but on our grants it was not commonplace for us, although Mr and Mrs Fishburn would take us there for a drink every week or two. Mrs Fishburn as well as being a lovely lady, was also an excellent cook. We therefore ate too much and although the menu was the same and predictable for the day of the week it was certainly enjoyable. Evening dinners and Sunday lunch were included in the price of our digs, and we therefore nearly always took them unless we were involved in some sporting event elsewhere.

And so to the local church in Bramley I went on my first Sunday. Needless to say there were attractive ladies within the congregation, and there was a meeting time and place afterwards. I cannot remember whether it was my first week, but certainly within a week or two I had met Kate Norfolk who was in the sixth form at the local grammar school, and interestingly had recently spent a term in an American school on an exchange scholarship. Kate lived with her parents at the other end of Bramley. Her father owned a company which ran a fleet of lorries. On my very first time visiting the house to collect Kate he said,

"Do borrow my car any time you wish." Unfortunately I had no driving licence. Over the next few months Kate and I became very good friends. One thing that Kate introduced me to was giving a talk to the sixth form of her school. I had had no previous experience and an audience of some 200 girls was very frightening. But apparently I entertained them sufficiently about my expedition to Arctic Lapland. She herself had been a junior athlete of some repute. I heard later that she married a medical student and they moved overseas.

With the money from an extra scholarship that the Drapers' Company awarded me I bought a 350cc Royal Enfield Motorcycle and used it every day to travel the four miles to the university. (Bancroft's School was a Worshipful Company of Drapers foundation). This could be quite exciting on icy days, and also on foggy days which were very common before the Clean Air Act was passed. As a motorcyclist one had better vision than car drivers and one very foggy day when driving home I had a stream of cars following my tail light. I turned into the long drive of my digs, and they all followed! It took some time to sort out the chaos. On future occasions I did prevent recurrences by stopping before the last turn.

As well as sailing, other sports became a very important part of my life. Badminton was the most important and I went straight into the university men's and mixed doubles teams. My mixed doubles partner was Dilys Hill. She had started life as a radiographer and had then become a sociology student. (She finished up as a professor). When practice finished on a Wednesday evening the union hop allowed free entry, and Dilys – who had been a gold medal ballroom dancer – taught me to dance, and also became my girlfriend.

Dancing also occurred at Balls organised by the union or various societies which included the Engineering Society. One year, and I cannot now remember whether I had no girlfriend, or that I could not afford it, instead of going to the ball I was asked to look after the bands and performers. The star was the famous jazz clarinetist Acker Bilk. What was unusual was that my job that night was to kneel behind him and hold him up. I never determined whether it was alcohol or drugs that caused the problem, but he still played his clarinet superbly. The other performers were Dick Charlesworth and his City Gents. They were delightful company and were my introduction to appreciating trad jazz.

Then came other sports. I was introduced to squash in my first year and by my third year was in the team. I also played tennis – mainly for introduction to the ladies, but I never progressed beyond the second team, and I even played the odd game of rugby. I never returned to athletics, partly because when I started at Leeds my right wrist had not completely healed from the fracture that had occurred six months previously.

Having sorted out the important parts of my life, the academic side must be mentioned.

To give an indication of what it was like for the undergraduate in 1957, in my year of admission 20% of the students were thrown out after a year, and of the remaining 80% half got a general degree, and only half of us received an honours degree.

The teaching was by lectures of which there were two or three each morning, and then in the afternoons there were practical classes in the subjects that we were studying that year. One afternoon a week and Saturday afternoon was for sport. It was in fact a six morning week. At least I had been used to that at school, but it was a great surprise to very many of my fellow students that they would have to work on Saturday mornings.

In my first year there was a course which involved all of the general engineering students, and more specialist courses in organic and physical chemistry, in physics and both applied and pure mathematics which were shared with undergraduates in those subjects. But surprisingly there was also a general introductory course in economics and trade union law. There was also an introduction to chemical engineering, but it was very much an introduction.

Throughout one's life one remembers special teachers and lecturers – some because they were outstanding, and some because they were appalling. In Leeds I remember Mr (or was it Dr) Whitehouse who taught organic chemistry. An interesting man who was also a well respected church organist. The lecture theatre was semi-circular and tiered, and we all had a numbered seat in which we had to sit. Anyone absent was recorded. He had an assistant who prepared the demonstrations on the front bench and which were remarkable. There could be a green solution in a beaker which had been there for five minutes, and Mr Whitehouse would say,

"And that will now turn red." Which it did within a few seconds. He was once demonstrating the instability of nitrogen tri-iodide which only explodes if touched when dry. He and his assistant were bent over the wet preparation when a person in the audience exploded a paper bag. They both jumped backwards, and the comment came out instantly,

"I see somebody failed the course last year."

Five minutes later the real explosion occurred. He carried on lecturing as though nothing had happened as we all came back down to our seats from the air.

Another lecturer in that first year was a new Civil Engineering lecturer from Poland. We all had mock exams in all subjects in the second term, and as might be expected no one did any work for them as they had no input to our final results.. The lecturer was extremely worried by our appalling results, and obviously thought that it was his fault. He then told us the questions in the paper at the end of that year which did count towards our finals. I understand that he was somewhat upset when we all got firsts, and that the next year students had a much tougher time.

One of the really outstanding lecturers that I have ever heard was Mr McRae. He lectured on coal science, and could come into a lecture room with two hundred engineering undergraduates and hold up his hand, and there would be total silence. I discovered later that he would practice each lecture in his room for an hour before the presentation. A remarkable and interesting man. The other lecturer that did leave an impression on me was Dr Bunn who was an excellent teacher in the physical chemistry laboratories.

A requirement of the scholarship that I had been awarded was that I worked in industry for six weeks during each summer vacation. These could be organised by me, or the university would help. The recommendation for my first summer was that I spent the period in a normal engineering workshop, and I therefore organised to go daily to the North Thames Gas Board at their Beckton works in East London. The problem was travelling from home, and I did this at the beginning on my motorcycle, and then found that two of the engineers lived quite close to me which enabled me to share their Bond Three-Wheeler – with me in the very small back. I learned to use lathes, planes and drills, and also some blacksmithing, which was the hardest work of all that I did. I also spent time in the drawing office. I still regret not having had a suitable camera as the men filling and emptying the horizontal retorts that produced the town gas with the flames, heat and fumes around were an amazing sight.

The second summer the suggestion was that I worked with a coke oven or iron manufacturing unit. One had always assumed that this would have to be up north, but incredibly the Ford Motor Company at Dagenham had both on site. I discovered that the reason for this was a policy of Fords that they should not be reliant on outside suppliers. The only necessity of materials coming in therefore was for coal and iron ore, which both came up the River Thames by barge. It was a fascinating six weeks finding out how industry worked before any car was actually made. I did spend some time in the engine manufacturing plant out of interest and my conclusion at the end was how awfully repetitive was that work. In many factories conversation between the workers was a major source of relief from boredom, but that was not possible because of the intensity of the manufacturing noise. I remember one job that I was asked to do, and still cannot believe that my calculations were not checked. A new gas holder had been built and when the gas from the coke oven filled it the large piston inside went up – but then would not come down as the density of coal gas is less than that of air. I was asked to calculate what extra weight needed to be put on the piston for it to work. I remember it being several tons and this, in concrete blocks, was distributed across the surface of the piston. And thankfully it worked. My other memory was spending a considerable time, especially during lunches, being aboard one of the sailing barges which delivered materials and having long conversations with the skipper.

My final summer before graduating I applied to work for Shell Research which was attached to their Stanlow refinery on the north east side of the Wirral Peninsula in Cheshire. This was a competitive application from all universities in the United Kingdom, and twenty-one of us were selected to work in the refinery or in the research laboratories. The scholarship also included board and lodging in a hotel in Chester and transport in and out each day.

It was a fascinating six weeks and I was involved in some interesting research. Shell had discovered that some of their refinery plant was rotting and collapsing for no obvious or expected reason. My small part of the lab was trying to find out, firstly why, and then what could be done to prevent the problem. The answer was that because the temperature of the reaction within the vessel had been increased there was a higher conversion of sulphur dioxide to sulphur trioxide, and this caused much greater corrosion to occur. The other very interesting research that was happening in the lab along the corridor was necessary as town gas made from coal for use in homes and industry was about to be replaced with natural gas from oil wells. Natural gas has no innate smell and it was necessary to invent a smell to put into the natural gas so that leaks could be detected by the user. The problem is a major challenge. The gas added must not be poisonous either when added or after burning. It must not block pipes or valves when hot or cold. It must be detectable by all people, identifiable and ideally not too unpleasant. We were the guinea pigs. The danger of having no smell became evident to me during the Bosnian war many years later when several explosions and injuries occurred. This is described in my book *'Plastic Surgery in Wars, Disasters and Civilian Life'*. One unrelated thing of interest was that despite the great competition between the oil companies and particularly the cheaper versions such as Jet Fuels, the tankers from all the companies, including Jet, came to the refinery to fill up. Interesting.

It would be interesting to know how many of the twenty-one of us finished up working for Shell.

I mentioned earlier about the BCRA conferences. It was normal to have a trade unionist as one of the speakers and in 1961 it was Frank Cousins, then General Secretary of the Transport and General Workers Union. I was asked to chair that session which was at my third conference. Mr Cousins gave his

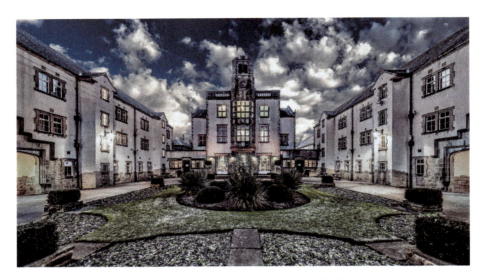

1.2 Devonshire Hall, University of Leeds in which I spent my third year. Designed on the basis of an Oxbridge college.

presentation and I asked for questions. There were about six and Mr Cousins was taking a very long time on the first. I manged to move him on, and his parting remark was to congratulate me. As I remember his words were.

"Congratulations – anyone who can shut me up is going to be going far!" Without specifying in which direction.

At Leeds University there were very few nationally famous scientists. Forty years earlier there had been Sir William and his son Lawrence Bragg who were Nobel laureates in Physics, and when I was at Cambridge (Chapter 4) I went out with a neice of William Bragg. One renowned scientist in post when I was at Leeds was the chemist Professor Dainton FRS, and by chance I went out with his daughter in Oxford (Chapter 6).

Finally accommodation. Perhaps 50% of undergraduates at Leeds lived at home. I mentioned earlier my marvellous digs in which I lived for two years, As well as sport we also shared an Austin 7 Chummy car which started my driving career. At the end of my second year I applied, and was selected to go to Devonshire Hall for the next academic year. Probably only 10-15% of men managed to obtain a place in a hall of residence, and Devonshire was the best known and of course the best! (Photo 1.2). An interesting building designed in 1928 on the pattern of Oxbridge colleges with individual staircases. It was situated in Headingly about 1 mile north of the university. I spent the first term in an annexe before moving into the main Hall. My last friend from there, another engineer, George Duffett died only a few months ago. We had an excellent tennis team with one ex junior Wimbledon player, and a swimming team that broke several university records (Chapter 17).

One marvellous story had been that John Stork, (Chapter 21), had his father up for some function. He introduced his father to the Warden, Cdr Evans ex Royal Navy Education Branch.

"Mr Evans, Mr Stork."

A cough or two from the Warden, and then,

"It's actually Cdr Evans."

And from John,

"Very sorry sir, Admiral Stork."

In my final year I moved into a flat on Woodhouse Moor, and even when over 21 years old, I still needed my mother's permission. Life has changed.

TWO

UNIVERSITY OF CAMBRIDGE – RESEARCH

I am not now sure why I even applied to go to Cambridge. I thought the chances of getting there were virtually nil, and I would have been happy to stay for a PhD at Leeds. In my final year as an undergraduate there was always in the background the challenge of moving to Cambridge. I think that I had had the inspiration for the move during the sailing matches that I had been involved in against Cambridge, and the Department of Chemical Engineering there was well established and world famous.

Having had the British Coke Research Association scholarship I worked for them for the three months at their research centre in Chesterfield which I needed to complete my scholarship requirement. (Photo 2.1). Bob Oxtoby and I were the two remaining BCRA fellows at Leeds and we went together to Chesterfield for our three months of work. We stayed with Mrs Dunn, the mother of my old digs mate Roger and

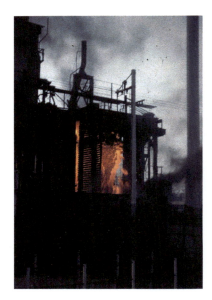

2.1 The Experimental Coke Oven at the British Coke Research Association, Chesterfield.

travelled across the city every day. We met the director Dr R A Mott who was acknowledged as the world expert on the coking industry, and he gave us the project of calculating the heat balance of their research coke oven. Surprisingly it had not been done before, but as we worked away at the solution the reason became obvious. It was a difficult challenge which often required putting estimates into the calculations, and also needing to work 24hr days on occasions to obtain valid readings. We eventually did solve the problem, and Dr Mott was suitably satisfied with the result. An interesting time, but not something that I wanted for my life work, and certainly not something that I would go into as a manager. Both Bob and I did leave the industry when I moved to medicine and Bob to education.

The exact order of what happened next I do not exactly remember, but after discussions in London I went to the headquarters of the National Coal Board (NCB) research station, which somewhat inappropriately was based in Cheltenham, and had a long and interesting interview with Dr Jacob Bronowski, the director of research. He was then a well-known television presenter of scientific programmes. Suddenly to be shown in to see him was an interesting and unexpected side issue of my visit to Cheltenham. He was interested in using fluidised beds to produce town gas from coal. The exact process was to make the coal dust with a hot gas flowing through it release the gas. By chance one of the sub departments of the chemical engineering department in Cambridge had been working on fluidised beds for some years, and he said that he would be willing to finance the scholarship at Cambridge (not personally – but through the NCB). The research is discussed later. I therefore went for an interview in the Department of Chemical Engineering in Cambridge, in effect carrying my own scholarship which I am sure made it much easier, and I was offered a place, and also the formal offer of a Cambridge University Research Scholarship. Cambridge is unusual in that even as a research student you have to have both a place in a university department and also in a college to be able to register for a degree.

I therefore had a walk around Cambridge to decide to which college I wished to apply. Needless to say for its architectural brilliance my first choice was King's College, however I knew nothing really about it, specifically or in general. I therefore applied to the College and went for an interview with Dr Ziman who was the postgraduate admissions tutor and a physics fellow at Kings. We certainly did not get on very well, and I was not offered a place. Such is life. The only connections that I then had with anyone in Cambridge

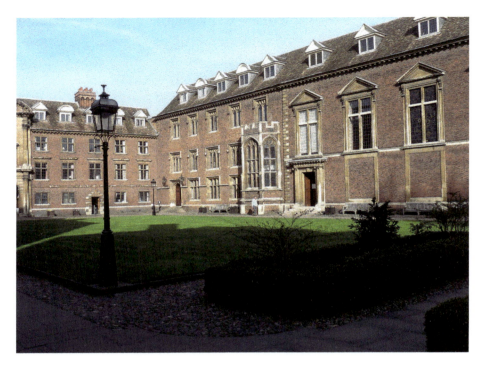

2.2 St Catharine's College, Cambridge. The College of which I was a member whilst doing research in Chemical Engineering.

was through sailing. I had competed against Cambridge on several occasions for Leeds, and was also involved through the British Universities Sailing Association. I therefore met some of my sailing colleagues in the Cambridge University Cruising Club clubhouse in Petty Cury for a cup of tea and found out considerably more about college life, and particularly that very few colleges had accommodation within the college for graduate students. This is now common throughout the university, and particularly with graduate colleges. But in 1961 graduate colleges did not exist and the colleges with accommodation were very rare. With this knowledge I applied to St Catharine's College and was accepted. (Photo 2.3). As it was late in the summer, the three rooms that were available in Silver Street for graduates were fully booked, and I therefore spent my first term in Girton. This sounds much more interesting than it in fact was, as my digs were in Girton village and not in Girton College (a lady's only college). It was always said of Girton girls that they had well developed thighs as they had to cycle some 3 miles out of the centre of town up almost the only Hill in

Cambridge to travel from the University to the College. Girton village is even further out than Girton College and I certainly did develop suitable thighs over that term.

And now a word about Cambridge. It was firstly completely different from Leeds for an undergraduate, and somewhat different for a post-graduate. Half the undergraduate teaching was done in the University, and half in one's college in supervisions with only 2 to 4 people for one hour for each subject in each week. And the undergraduates were different as well. In those days in 1961 one could almost divide the undergraduates into three groups. A third were academically brilliant, a third were good sportsmen, and a third were something else. This included acting, music or even as one friend of mine told me – playing tiddlywinks for England. I do have to add that he did get a first class degree in physics and a PhD afterwards. There were also a considerable number of undergraduates who had 'connections', either through schools, parents or through other means which very particularly obtained by the sons of fathers from a college. The majority of these latter undergraduates were in groups two and three, but some were without doubt also academically brilliant. This academically brilliant group were very different from Leeds. Compared with school I had been disappointed by the academic level of most of the students in Leeds, but in Cambridge in 1961 I had more than met my match. The other thing that was completely different at Cambridge (and Oxford of the other universities) was the shortage of places for women students. There were just three colleges out of the twenty-two that then existed which admitted women, making about 10% of the University undergraduates female, and of course there were then no mixed colleges at all. It is also an interesting thought that in 1961 only approximately 3% of students in England went on from school to university. Things were changing with the foundation of new Universities, and in this period Sussex, Kent, East Anglia, Essex, York and several others had just been founded or were in the process of being founded.

The research students were a different group. Compared with about seven or eight thousand undergraduates there were about twelve hundred research students. Perhaps one half of these had been graduates from Cambridge, and the other half were taken from universities throughout Britain and from all over the world. As well as research students, virtually all of whom were doing a PhD, there were also postgraduate students in education, divinity, music, architecture and medicine who were not working for a PhD but for another higher qualification.

In 1961 all of the colleges took undergraduate and postgraduate students. The one anomaly was Fitzwilliam College whose students were mostly postgraduate and studying to teach. These students were able to study within the University without being a full member of the University. The first postgraduate college was Darwin College, founded in 1964 in the house of Gwen Raverat a member of the Darwin family, and a famous author who wrote the lovely book 'Period Piece'.

One's contacts as a research student at university are very different to those that one makes as an undergraduate. Firstly the research, where by far the most important contact is with one's supervisor. My supervisor was Dr David Harrison – later Sir David. In our first meeting he told me the requirements that the National Coal Board required.

The experiment, which was unique, was to study a fluidised bed, normally used for the excellent heat transfer characteristics of beds, but in which a chemical reaction was also occurring. This was what would be happening if town gas was being produced from coal particles within a bed. The NCB had also determined that the minimum size at which the experiment would be conducted was a bed of 25cm in diameter. I therefore went to the library to do some research and produced engineering drawings for the apparatus which had a reaction chamber of 25cm diameter. With help from the department workshop the necessary parts and instruments were ordered, and construction slowly began. At this point I should have noticed that the internal diameter of all the other similar experiments in the department were never larger than 5cm, and it did indeed turn out that the semi-industrial scale at which I was working was impractical for a university project with a single inexperienced research student.

It is possible that several research students are working on similar projects, but unfortunately this was not the case for my work. I had a small amount of help from other academics which was mostly about statistics. My main help came from the workshop staff when I was struggling to construct and make function the large complicated experiment that I had had to design and build. Looking back, I think Dr Harrison and I both let each other down to some extent. I was far too inexperienced to realise, and to say, that the experiment was not working, and I think that was also true for Dr Harrison. Within the department Dr John F Davidson (later Professor Davidson FRS) who has been described as the Father of Fluidisation had an active team of research fellows working under his supervision, I had contact with all of these in the laboratory, but none were working on a project close to mine. Towards the end of my first year I had to submit a report of my progress, and this was accepted with no problems and my registration for a PhD was confirmed. I would however say that at that time the apparatus was still being completed and had not been turned on.

Within the department was a new computer and it was obvious to us all that its use would aid our research. It was an IBM 1620 computer with a memory of 10k – far less than a simple modern watch. It was in an air conditioned room, and the construction was with semiconductors and valves. It would normally spend at least half a day a week being serviced or repaired. We had to learn to write our own programmes, and a simple one would take all night to run, and when it went wrong in the middle of the night it would produce a large amount of waste paper. Definitely a challenge, but very worthwhile as I was to discover over the next years.

The research went slowly with problems obtaining the equipment and with the construction. I therefore became involved in supervising physical chemistry in my College, and physics in the world famous Cavendish Laboratory which was next to our department in Pembroke Street. One day I was having a break in the Cavendish tearoom when an elderly gentleman came up to me and asked me what I was doing. I explained and he said that I must meet one of his colleagues to see if any help could be offered. The person who had approached me was Prof P A M Dirac the Nobel Prize winning Lucasian Professor of Mathematics. The undergraduate teaching in the laboratories was very interesting, as were the other demonstrators and the undergraduates. I specialised in heat, electricity and light and also radioactivity at a very basic level. This could be amusing. We would warn the student about the radioactive substance that they were experimenting with, and they would take extreme care to keep it as far away as possible. At the end of the experiment we would then hold their watch, of which the majority in those days had radioactive paint for illumination, under the Geiger counter, and the activity was always much greater than the experiment had produced. I also remember a pair of young lady students who put together the electrical circuit that was needed. Nothing worked. So I suggested they did it again as there must be something wrong. On the third go I gave up, and pointed out that if they turned on the switch on the wall all would work perfectly. I took one of these out one evening and was walking down King's Parade with her when we were approached by a 'bulldog'. The Cambridge 'bulldog' is very different to a normal bulldog. They are paid staff who accompany the University Proctor whose duty is to see that the students behave and follow the university rules. The particular 'bulldog' coming over was one of the Cavendish laboratory staff and obviously recognised us both. In my second year in Cambridge graduate students did not have to wear a gown at night, but undergraduates still did. The lass with me was not wearing her gown. Our technician politely asked me if I was a member of the university, and I formally told him that I was a graduate. He then went back to the Proctor on the other side of the road and appraised him of the situation – but without mentioning my companion. She escaped a fine, and thanked him profusely the following day.

The other work that I did was to teach "O" level mathematics in the Cambridge Technical College for two hours a week. To get into my particular class the students had failed the exam at least twice previously. Some were a challenge. Many were on day release and totally uninterested. Some had no understanding of mathematics – or of much else – and about half actually wanted or needed the exam. I came to an agreement that if they were not interested they would sit quietly in the back of the room and do whatever they liked. It was the easiest teaching that I have ever done as I needed no preparation at all. And I did get 50% through. The following year I went back to do the same course, but they were obviously short elsewhere and asked me to teach student cooks general science. I asked for a copy of the syllabus and previous exam papers, and was told that neither existed – but they just had to have two hours of general science a week. After some thought I decided that heat transfer would be useful for cooks and started teaching that. The situation was made much worse as some of the class had "O" level physics, but most had never even heard of the subject. By the end of the second week I realised that they and I were in trouble together and suggested that the next week they could ask me any question about science, and I would either answer it then, or the following week. A marvellous and lucky solution, and suddenly I had an interested group of students. Half the questions were on cosmology or similar which I could answer straight away, and the other half on medicine. These latter I mostly had to look up, and I do wonder whether this work contributed to my later change to medicine.

On the social side one made friends amongst one's research colleagues and with other colleagues in sports and other interests. In Cambridge and Oxford there were also contacts within one's college. One interesting social contact

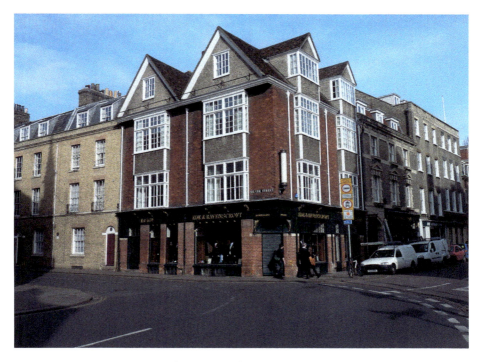

2.3 No 1 Silver Street The post graduate rooms.
My room was on the second floor on the corner.

which arose from my Tech teaching was a party in someone's flat where one person sat on the floor and talked or replied to nobody. I found out later that it was Tom Sharpe, who had just been thrown out of South Africa for anti-apartheid work and was clearly very depressed. He later became the famous author who wrote, amongst many other books, the Wilt series of novels.

Within the department we were a close knit team, particularly in each admission year. This was partly by subject but much more by all working in the same laboratories. My particular friends Leo Pyle and Tony Gillham were also in the same college, and Tony and I occupied two of the three graduate rooms in No 1 Silver Street (Photo 2.3). The third person in No 1 was Martin Gardner who was doing a one year course in statistics. When he left he was replaced by a very quiet American. Trying to make contact Tony and I invited him in for a drink.

"Coffee or Horlicks," asks Tony.

"What is Horlicks?" was the question. He decided to try this and was then asked whether he would like sugar added. This was put in.

He drank it very slowly and when Tony asked what he thought of the new drink his reply was,

"It's very salty isn't it?" Tony had added two large spoonfuls of salt – and for some reason we never became close friends with the American, who we were convinced thought that he had done it deliberately.

Tony was different to the rest of us and was definitely a hunting shooting and beagling man. He remained as a chemical engineer and became a very successful businessman and now lives in Yorkshire. Leo was a much more typical Cambridge post-graduate. He had a measured IQ of more than 180 – a true genius level. He also remained as a chemical engineer and became a professor at Reading University. However obviously becoming bored writing his thesis he also wrote a book on Catholic theology which was published in the same month. After retiring to the Lake District he fell off a mountain and was sadly killed. The third person in the group was Charles Everett who had come from Manchester University with Leo. Charles went to work in the United States and then returned to a Fellowship in Downing College before dying far too young with a brain malignancy. Hank Schleinitz was an American from MIT with whom I shared a house for my final year, and he also introduced me to ice hockey. John Pittman has remained a close friend. We were the two in our year that did not complete our PhDs in Cambridge. John then moved to Imperial College for further research and did complete a PhD before becoming a lecturer at Swansea University. A remarkable number of the students did remain within universities and became professors in England, Australia, America and India. The most remarkable of all was Max Richards who was two years senior to me. He returned to Trinidad as professor in chemical engineering and then became Chancellor of the University and finally President of his country, Trinidad and Tobago.

On the social side within the department we had a cricket team that played in a 20 over evening league within the departments of the university, and which included academic and technical staff and postgraduate students. With the help of Dr Turner, an old Cambridge blue and Dave Sutherland of my year, a remarkable Australian cricketer who averaged over 100 in all forms of cricket one year, we were champions for two years. There was a South African the year below us who we will not forget. One evening we were all at a drinks party in Pembroke College and whilst we were inside it snowed quite heavily. As we came out he took one look at the snow and started rolling in it. A rude word came out and then the comment,

"It's cold!". What he was expecting we never did discover. Many years later I met him in South Africa where he was employed by the company of a friend of mine. The world is a small place.

Most of my close friends within college were through sport and these are mentioned in the relevant sections of Part 3. However I was involved in helping with the statistics of one friend Charles Higham, now a very well known archaeologist and living in New Zealand. When it became too complicated for me, I introduced him to Chris Petrie who was the outstanding mathematician in our year.

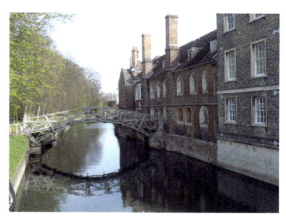

2.4 The Backs. Queen's College on the right and Newton's Mathematical Bridge in the centre.

Within college there was a middle common room for postgraduates. We ate together once a week in College, and the room which was situated in the oldest part of college, was available at any time. There was contact between each of us and our own research supervisors but when I was living in Silver Street, on the floor above were two fellows Drs John Shakeshaft and David Smith. In conversation with them I suggested having a monthly meeting in an evening of the more junior fellows and the PhD students. Over a bottle or two of port each fellow or student would take it in turns to present their work for one hour, and this was followed by a questions session. These were very popular and made an enormous contribution to college academic life. There was one occasion that was somewhat different. We were due to meet in the room of Dr Alfred Maddock. He was a very well known inorganic chemist working with radioactivity. He was also well known to be considerably forgetful. It was said that his lab had originally been down several steps. By the time he had deposited quantities of radioactive materials which had had to be covered with layers of concrete, his lab was up several steps. On the occasion of the particular meeting we all stood around with no sign of Alfie. Eventually John Shakeshaft phoned him at home.

"Are you supposed to be somewhere?"

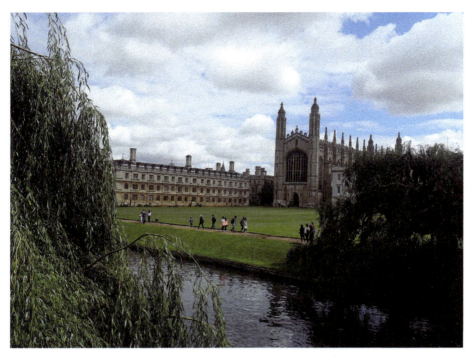

2.5 The Backs with King's College to the right and Clare College to the left.

"Yes," was the reply, "where?"

He arrived soon with several bottles of port – and was of course forgiven.

A phenomenal three years with many lasting friends and memories in a very beautiful city (Photos 2.4 and 2.5). And young ladies have not even been mentioned. Although rare, they existed, and will be written about in the chapter on my bachelorhood in a later book.

THREE

THE CHEMICAL ENGINEER

My final term doing research at Cambridge was less than satisfactory. The size of the experiment which had been set at 25 cm in diameter by the National Coal Board was, looking back, a completely impractical piece of work for an inexperienced PhD student. As I said earlier this had been a requirement of Dr Jacob Bronowski for the scholarship and had unfortunately been agreed by my supervisor Dr David Harrison. What was becoming increasingly clear was that the experimental error was greater than the effect for which I was looking.

The other problem which was also becoming more apparent was that the original need of the research to discover how to produce Town Gas from coal was becoming less and less important. Two things were happening simultaneously, firstly Town Gas production and use was in decline both because of the danger to human life from Town Gas inhalation, and also the damage to the atmosphere, particularly from the sulphur and the nitrogen oxide gasses produced, was becoming more apparent. At the same time natural gas was becoming more and more relevant as the future source of domestic gas. It was being imported from elsewhere before the first North Sea oil field was discovered in 1964 and production began here in 1967. There were problems with natural gas, one of which was that it had no natural distinctive smell, and by chance in the laboratories which were next to me whilst I had been working at the Thornton Research Centre for Shell the development of this smell was being carried out, and we were used as the guinea pigs. (Chapter 1).

I was therefore in a position with research which was not submittable for a Cambridge PhD, and a scholarship that was running out, and may well not have been renewed as the research became less relevant to the National Coal Board. I therefore started looking for employment and came across an advertisement for an assistant lecturer post in the chemical engineering department of the proposed University of Surrey for which the salary would be £1,400 a year. I applied for this and was successful in my interview, about which I remember nothing. Clearly my annual research reports and references had been sufficient.

A brief introduction to the background of the university is of interest, and also explained over the next two or three years some of the successes and failures both of the chemical engineering department and of the whole university. Harold Wilson, as Prime Minister, decided to expand the university base in Great Britain, and in particular to expand the technological universities by converting the ten Colleges of Advanced Technology which then existed into universities. This included the Battersea College of Technology which had been founded in 1891 as the Battersea Polytechnic Institute (Photo 3.1), with the aim of 'giving higher education for the poorer inhabitants of London'. In

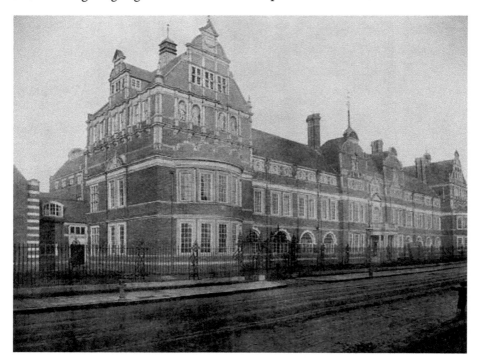

3.1 The Battersea Polytechnic College. Later to become the first College of Advanced Technology and then the University of Surrey. I lectured there for three years.

1956 it was renamed as the Battersea College of Advanced Technology, and was the first CAT in Great Britain. It was then incorporated with a Polish University which had come to Britain after the war and had been based in Putney. Battersea was different to the other nine Harold Wilson instant universities in that, as well as the technological and science subjects offered, it also had good and large departments in music and in hotel catering. The plan for the next year or two was to have the relevant Act of Parliament passed to establish it as an independent university, the University of Surrey, and then to build the new University in Guildford. This was also unique in that the other nine universities kept their original names, and remained in the towns or cities in which they had been established. Therefore in my first year there it was formally known as the Battersea College of Advanced Technology (proposed University of Surrey). It was at that time a college of the University of London, and in that first year the degree course and examinations were of the University of London and external London degrees were awarded. The Department of Chemical Engineering had been in existence for several years and I joined the academic staff of seven other members under the leadership of Dr (later Prof) S R Tailby. The second most senior member of the staff was in fact one of the Polish lecturers, Dr Potalski. The remainder of the Department were Dr WJ Thomas, Dr Ernest Clutterbuck, Dr Roy Goulcher, Frank Moles and Arnold Freedman. In the first two academic years there were some 30 to 40 undergraduate students who came in with their relevant advanced level examinations. In the third year however these were joined by another 20 or 30 graduate students who had degrees either in chemistry or in engineering, and were converting to become chemical engineers. Many of these were from overseas, and in particular India, but some were also from other universities in Great Britain, or were graduates of Battersea CAT. There were also three or four PhD students and also some older students who had come in from industry with a Higher National Diploma qualification to obtain a degree. Many of these were older than me and all of them had more experience of industry than myself, and also of the majority of our academic staff.

In most respects the college was already acting as a university. There were lectures and laboratory and workshop practicals. What however was somewhat different to many older and established universities was that the majority of the students lived at home or in flats. There were only two halls of residence.

I started in September 1964 and was sent on two separate courses on university teaching methods. Both as an undergraduate and as a postgraduate

I had of course been to a multitude of lectures of considerable variability of style and ability. The two courses on which I was sent were interestingly very different. The first course was for all new science, technology and engineering lecturers in the University of London who were starting that same year. There was very little that was new in this course, but the most stressful part of it was that we all had to give a 10 minute lecture stating what we were trying to teach, and at what level – in other words first, second or third year students. I do not remember what my lecture was on, but I was enormously cheered up when Leo Pyle, who had been with me in my department in Cambridge and had just been appointed to Imperial College was also on the course. Leo, who was one of the two most intelligent people that I have ever known well, rather messed it up by giving a two-hour lecture in 10 minutes at a speed which was completely inappropriate and almost inaudible, and at the wrong academic level. Needless to say being Leo, he very rapidly learned from his experience. The second course was very different. It was based at the Roehampton College of Education and was for all of the new lecturers in all subjects at the University of Surrey. There were two things I remember well about that course. The first was a lecturer who came in and said that the art of lecturing was to include in each lecture three things. Information, humour, and surprise. The examples he gave remain with me to this day and were an incredibly useful introduction. The second lecture that I still remember, and would love to have the courage to repeat, was somebody (a brilliant actor) who came in and for a quarter of an hour did it all wrong. He walked up and down, he muttered at the board, he wrote so that one couldn't read it, threw his keys in the air and did all those things one knew one should not do. He then went on to a monotone, and talked rapidly for five minutes. He stopped, looked around at all twenty of us and said,

"What was I talking about?" Not surprisingly none of us knew. It was the most brilliant demonstration of how not to lecture, and therefore any time afterwards whenever I started doing any of those things, I said to myself – stop – I must not do this. And after my three days of instruction on how to lecture, and how to teach practicals, I was considered a suitably trained university lecturer. I still don't understand why it takes a full year to train a schoolteacher!

And so to London. I had arranged to share a flat in Earls Court with two trainee accountants that I had met through a sailing connection on the Isle of Wight. I then arrived at the University to meet members of my department and very luckily to be given a room of my own. I was taken into the senior common room for a cup of tea and immediately came across a very close ex-colleague of mine. Graham Taylor had been in my form at school where we were both scientists. He was also a fellow Scout in my troop, and we had sailed together and against each other for many years – he as captain of London University Sailing Club and myself as captain of Leeds University Sailing Club, and by incredible chance had both been selected in the same British Universities team to sail against the French universities (Chapter 21). He had joined the University of Surrey a year before me as a lecturer in electronic engineering.

My duties in that first year were remarkably light. I was teaching reaction kinetics and advanced heat transfer as my two lecture course subjects. However I discovered that it would take me nearly two days of work to produce a one hour lecture. Needless to say when one was starting one was extremely worried that one could not answer any questions that were asked during or after the lecture. Therefore a large amount of background reading was necessary to help with my relaxation before each lecture. I was also teaching in the engineering laboratory for, if I remember correctly, three three-hour periods a week.

For the first few months I was still travelling back at weekends to Cambridge to be sure that my research project could not usefully continue. I stayed with old friends Dick Hardy, David Brooks and Greg Sage in their flat besides Parker's Piece. Also sharing that flat on occasions was Winston Tubman and his wife. Winston was the nephew of the President of Liberia. A very interesting couple. Regrettably Winston failed in his later bid to follow his uncle as President.

In London I set up a research project related to the work I had been doing in Cambridge. It was based on a much smaller size experiment. I was still registered for my PhD in Cambridge, but it became clear after some months of work that even the modified project was not viable to produce useful, reproducible results. Within the University I became involved both with the badminton and the squash clubs, and joined the Conservative Association who promptly made me their President. They were clearly short of candidates as then and now most universities are strongly left-wing.

In the west end of London through my new flatmates, and through other contacts a social life rapidly grew. Within the university I had some social life with my old friend Graham Taylor, and also began to have a closer friendship with Ernest Clutterbuck, who had a sense of humour close to my own. Looking back it is interesting that at no point did I ever have an invitation to a meal with my professor or any fellow lecturers in my department with the exception of Ernest. This was so so different to life in Cambridge where a large amount of social contact between students and staff was normal, but unfortunately very similar to that at Leeds, where again it had been totally absent. There was an occasional social function. I remember one cocktail party in the senior common room. I was going on to a rather posh do in London afterwards and was dressed in white tie and tails and standing near the entrance. And in walked the Vice-chancellor, Dr Leggett, who looked at me somewhat embarrassed and apologised for not having read his invitation. I, also embarrassed, explained why I was so dressed, and we then had an interesting conversation – the first that I had had with him. Another regular semi-social occasion did occur because the university had a Department of Hotel Catering, and as part of this served very excellent three course lunches every day during terms in their restaurant to give them experience. These were open to members of the academic staff and their guests for five shillings – but unfortunately without wine. The positive side was the food, the negative side was that they took a minimum of an hour which was a large slice of the day, but that was almost the only place to meet one's colleagues socially. And the third opportunity for a social occasion was to be taken out for a lunch by visiting company interviewers who were recruiting our graduates. It was a time when industry was doing well and there was a severe shortage of qualified chemical engineers. The companies therefore invited one or two of us to an excellent lunch to find out which of our prospective graduates we recommended before the interviews started. I am not sure what the alcohol level was during the interviews! And so the year progressed with no very clear future developing in front of me.

Towards the end of that first year however there was an advertisement within the university for an academic warden at one of the two halls of residence. It was suggested that I might apply for this. I did and after a competitive interview, was appointed. That summer I returned to Sea View Yacht Club as assistant secretary and a sailing instructor. I also gave up my position in the flat knowing that I would be returning to the Hall.

The larger of the two halls that the university owned was on the west side of Battersea Park. It was a multi-storey, relatively modern building and was for male students only. There was a warden and two assistant wardens. My hall of residence was a very much more interesting building. It was situated on North Side, Clapham Common. From the university one went up Queenstown Road, which half way up changed its name to Cedars Road and as this hit North Side, Clapham Common, on the left and the right were two magnificent large

Victorian buildings of four or five stories each. These two buildings had been constructed for the heads of state who were visiting the 1851 exhibition in London. In 1964 the building to the west had been converted into flats, and the building to the east was the Hall of Residence. What was very unusual about that Hall, apart from its magnificent building, was that it was mixed sex. In 1964 this was a great rarity among university halls of residence anywhere, and the only exceptions I knew were the accommodation halls at some medical schools. There was a domestic warden, a lovely lady who was about 60, and myself as the academic warden. We had, as I remember it, 132 mostly first year students, with a slightly larger number of males than females. I was allocated two rooms, a sitting room/study and a single bedroom with a small bathroom, all on the first floor. I had no kitchen, and I was expected to eat with the students. In front was a car park which was extremely convenient when I needed to rebuild my car, and there were virtually no gardens. There was however, by going up onto the roof, the most magnificent view across the whole of London which, in those days before skyscrapers were built everywhere, was almost unmatched.

One of the first things that I did after long discussions with the Post Office was to convert its official address to the North Side Hall of Residence which I felt gave it a cachet that No 54 North Side did not. One of my duties, which could be interesting but often was not, was to have four students join me on the high table for dinner on two nights a week. These came by rota, and I also invited lecturers from throughout the university to improve the interest and to discover about some of my colleagues. Through these dinners I met and became friendly with Drs Brian and Catherine Reuben, a chemist and a linguist and John and Rita Weston, an accountancy lecturer and an excellent tennis player. And surprisingly I was given two bottles of sherry a week to entertain the visitors and the students to pre-dinner drinks. (The things that one remembers). These dinners were quite hard work, particularly when I did not have visiting lecturers. With few exceptions the intellectual interest of most of the students – and the hotel management students were the exception – did not go much further than soccer or another sport. And as soccer had never been an interest of mine this could make the dinner conversation somewhat difficult. The students were all sharing rooms, either between two or four of them, and the sexes were separated on different floors. I am sure that sexual encounters did go on, but they were surprisingly not very obvious. One of the more useful things that I did do was to offer weekly supervisions in either chemistry or physics to small groups of the students. I started with the chemical engineering students, and the information spread to students from other relevant departments who were in the Hall. I was asked if I could do the same for them. These were clearly based on the supervisions that occurred in Cambridge and became surprisingly popular and well attended, and I hope useful.

In my second year, life in the Department had changed very little at the beginning, but the new special subject of biochemical engineering was being introduced to various departments in universities throughout the country. I was asked to prepare to take on the task of teaching this the following year. Apart from an interest in biology which had been lifelong, I had had no previous training at any level in a biological subject. After discussions it was decided that I would attend both biochemistry and microbiology courses with the first-year undergraduates. It must have been very strange for them to have a university lecturer with them. With my background in organic chemistry, the biochemistry was easy. However I found the microbiology absolutely fascinating and became very involved in it. As a further additional duty within the Department I was put in charge of admissions for the following year, but did not change or increase my lecture courses or the practical work in the laboratories.

There were many more students wanting to come to read chemical engineering than we had places. Much of the selection was done on the application forms, but I did interview the majority of the prospective students who lived in the UK. I well remember two particular interviews. The first was a young lad with an excellent application form with the exception of his headmaster's report which stated,

"I do not think this boy is worth a place at university this year, or at any year in the future."

Because of the information on the rest of his form I decided to interview this lad, and he gave an excellent interview. At the end of the interview, I said to him,

"You clearly did not get on well with your headmaster." He went a little red and said,

"No sir." I asked him if he could tell me why not. He went a little redder and then quietly said,

"I made his daughter pregnant." I gave him a place, and he went on to get a first class degree. The second lad I remember was an Indian and during the general conversation I asked him from where he came.

"B'a'sea."

This was not a place that I recognised in India, and I asked him to tell me in more detail.

"Battersea mate," was the answer. All very embarrassing, but in those days very few Indian lads had Cockney accents. Again I gave him a place and he also went on to get a first. A most delightful lad who prospered in the department and in my Hall, and I remember was extremely helpful to some less able students.

During that year it did however become clear to me that my lack of industrial experience made teaching undergraduate engineers more difficult. I had had four short periods in industry as an undergraduate and new graduate, but two of these were doing research which I had found very interesting, but less relevant when teaching. Sometime during that year therefore, and I do not remember how it happened, I applied to ICI to spend the summer vacation working for them. I was offered a post as a technical officer within the Agricultural Division which was based at Billingham in Teesside. This was both interesting and had the added advantage that it was very well paid. I was also given free accommodation in Norton Hall which was their excellent residential centre for unmarried senior staff.

I therefore drove up to Norton Hall in my old MG TC and the next day went into the incredibly smelly and old Billingham chemical plant. (Photo 3.2). At that time it was the largest chemical works in Europe. I really did not know what to expect but after a briefing was given a project. The manufacture of ammonia is mainly for agricultural use, and it is one of the most important chemical industrial processes both then and now. It is carried out at a high-pressure, and at a high temperature, which make the process both dangerous and very expensive in energy. One of the reasons for this expense is that the nitrogen

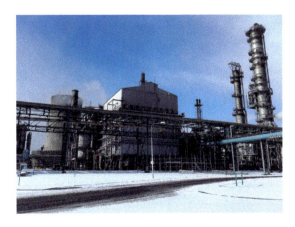

3.2 ICI Billingham. The Ammonia plant where I worked one summer designing a new ammonia plant which was later adopted.

Image courtesy of CF Fertilisers

is obtained from the atmosphere but always incorporates approximately 1% of inert gases. As the nitrogen is used up in the process, the aptly named inert gases build up within the reactor. To stop their concentration becoming too high they are continually bled off. This is wasteful in energy and hydrogen and also of the inert gases which themselves have some uses for different processes. A chemist in the laboratory had noticed that the inert gases were soluble in liquid ammonia. What was very unusual was that the gases became more soluble as the temperature of the liquid ammonia increased. This is completely contradictory to all other gas and liquid solutions. The question that I was given therefore was to find out if there was a possibility that a process and plant could be designed to use this new discovery, and whether it would be a cheaper and more efficient method of manufacture. The work that had been done in the laboratory was done at relatively low pressures and temperatures, and my final conclusion after three months of work was that further laboratory research was needed at higher temperatures and pressures, as it would only then be possible to estimate the outcome of the process if one had this further information. Needless to say the work was not published as it was very much a trade secret and I was sworn to secrecy. Many years later, and by complete chance, I met a senior ICI employee who told me that my method had gone into production and was being used.

I had only been there a couple of days and had taken a telephone call for my boss and left him a note on his desk. Very soon afterwards he appeared and asked who had left him the note. I thought that this was somewhat unusual but in conversation the reason for his worry became obvious. On his first day as an employee, he had been left a similar note. He had not checked its origin and had phoned the Chairman of ICI for a somewhat difficult conversation. Ever since he had checked the origin of any such request.

The division had just acquired three IBM 360 1MB computers at a cost of £1M each. Being IBM, the programming language was Fortran which I had used at Cambridge. The computing department had used Algol on their previous computers, and I would regularly have a telephone call asking me what to do. They very soon learnt themselves, as advising computer experts was definitely not my forte.

Those three months were a very interesting and fascinating time, and made me think quite seriously about applying to stay at ICI. Life in industry was different but not as different as I had imagined, particularly in the Research and Development Department.

There were however major disadvantages in the area in that the social life, apart from sailing with Dr Robin Steavenson every weekend (Chapter 21), drinking in Norton Hall with my colleagues and the occasional game of squash, was almost absent. Any young ladies in the area with any get up and go, got up and went to London leaving a distinct absence of normal life. Perhaps not the only reason, but I therefore returned to Battersea, still as Warden of North Side Hall of Residence and now promoted to a full lectureship with a salary of £1800 a year.

The hall had a new cohort of students all looking very nervous. The Department had changed in that Roy Goulcher had left to take up an appointment at the University of Lancaster as a mathematician rather than an engineer. And so my main problem at this stage was to organise the biochemical engineering option for which twelve third year students had signed up. As well as the course of lectures I also had to organise visits to various parts of the biochemical industry. These included discovering how penicillin was made, how beer was brewed, sewage was treated, and several visits into the food industry – both to Unilever research laboratories and to the actual plants making the food. The students were very keen, and we progressed very much together. The other courses that I was still giving were no great stress as by this time I was becoming a relatively experienced lecturer, and I also continued on with the admissions.

And then in that summer term of 1967 I made the decision to return to university to become a surgeon (Chapter 4). It was however almost as if chemical engineering wanted to keep me. I was invited by my old Cambridge colleague Leo Pyle to lunch at Imperial College where he was a lecturer. There must have been a previous conversation as after lunch I was taken to meet Professor Ernst Chain, the Nobel Prize Laureate with Fleming and Florey for their work on penicillin. Within Imperial College he had quite a sizeable biochemical engineering plant and he clearly wanted someone to run and develop it. After a long conversation he offered me a lectureship – basically as his assistant but with some biochemical engineering teaching. Having been turned down by Imperial as an undergraduate I was needless to say very flattered; but with my medical place at Cambridge, and also realising that Professor Chain clearly believed that there were twenty five working hours in each day, and that he would be a difficult person for whom to work, and the following day I politely declined his offer. And where I would now be if I had accepted it, I will never know. Having been accepted at Cambridge to read medicine, and having received a suitable scholarship, I finally made up my mind and resigned my lectureship. The other thing that happened in that same term was that I became engaged.

Chemical engineering did not quite finish there as in the summer of 1967 I moved down to stay in Ernest's self-constructed new house in Camberley and worked for the University helping them to move into their new building, and again doing all the department admissions. It was somewhat strange that a chemical engineer leaving the profession was asking the students why they wanted to go into the profession. I do not think that anyone discovered the anomaly. The other thing with which I became very involved during that summer was designing an analogue computer system to record the experiments in the engineering laboratories. This took a considerable amount of time, but when finished would probably have been the most innovative laboratory computer system in chemical engineering (or probably also chemistry or other engineering) at that time in Great Britain or perhaps anywhere. After the two months of hard work the Prime Minister Harold Wilson unfortunately withdrew the money for the project. And how little I know about computing now. One other possible future project was also discussed with a local research company which was using plasma physics for the study of some chemical reactions.

In my first year at Cambridge I also returned on some Friday afternoons to give the biochemical engineering lectures. This was of major psychological advantage to me as I would otherwise have found the sudden loss of responsibility very difficult.

And that was the end of my formal chemical engineering, a subject I found fascinating but could see very little future as an academic without a higher degree or research papers. So many other aspects of university life had become more important, and I also realised that my mathematics was not up to being a high-class academic engineer.

Part Two

Medicine and Plastic Surgery

FOUR

UNIVERSITY OF CAMBRIDGE – UNDERGRADUATE

Towards the end of 1966, I decided to look into the possibility of returning to university to read medicine. My memory is that this was a sudden decision, but friends have since told me that I had been talking about it for some months. At Bancroft's School biology was not taught – it was thought to be a girls' subject. And so, although I had a long term interest in natural history, I had no formal qualification in a biological subject.

I remember the events quite distinctly. On one Sunday early afternoon, I phoned Roger Tapp at Clare College in Cambridge. Roger and I had been very good friends during my postgraduate years in Cambridge. He was at that stage a lecturer in physiology, and also by chance involved in selecting medical students for Clare College. We discussed the problems of the lack of a biological subject and what I might have to do to fill in this gap. He said he would make some enquiries, which he did of Dr Gordon Wright, an anatomist and the senior fellow in the medical faculty at Clare College. Roger phoned me back that same evening and said that Clare College would offer me a place. Astonishment! I then asked about the problem with biology, and he said that they had decided that I could simply cover it during my first year as a medical student. Out of courtesy he would tell St Catharine's, my old college. On the Tuesday morning I received a letter from St Catharine's requiring me to go for an interview that same afternoon. I duly went up to Cambridge for a discussion with Dr Comline, who was a veterinary physiologist and the Fellow in charge of medical admissions to the college. His first question and in a somewhat gruff tone was.

"Why did you apply to Clare College?"

I told him what had happened, and that I had not actually applied to Clare College. He immediately said that I was coming back to St Catharine's and that was the end of the discussion. I understood later from Roger that he had threatened Clare that there would not be sufficient places in the physiology laboratory, which Dr Comline organised, for all Clare students if I had gone to Clare rather than going back to my old college. Looking back it was very nice to be wanted, but I was much less impressed at the time.

The next problem was acquiring funding. I had saved up a reasonable amount of my lecturer's salary whilst at the University of Surrey, and I also considered joining the military. It turned out that the military did not fund undergraduates to read medicine *ab initio*, but they would be very happy to fund me as soon as I had passed my second MB examination at the end of the second year. I therefore looked for other possibilities and discovered that the London County Council had a small number of highly sought-after scholarships which they awarded to people who were already graduates, but who wanted to transfer either to medicine or to divinity. I duly applied for one of these scholarships. My main referee was Dr D M A Leggett, the Vice Chancellor of the University of Surrey. I am still not sure whether he did this out of the goodness of his heart, or because he wanted to get rid of me from the staff at the University of Surrey! In fact he must have said very polite and nice things about me. I had a short interview and was duly awarded a scholarship which would start that September (1967) and last me for the full five years. And so back to St Catharine's.

Whilst I had been at Cambridge having my interview at my old college, I dropped in to see my old Department of Chemical Engineering, and in particular Margaret Sansome who was the secretary to Professor Danckwerts. Margaret had been a good friend during my three years of research at Cambridge and she asked me where I was going to stay when I came back, to which I had no answer. She said there was a spare room in her house if I would like to use it. She also offered it to me at a very, very, reasonable rate and having had a look at it, I knew that I would be very happy to move in there. So one problem solved. She also made it clear that she would be very happy for my fiancé, Moira, to come and stay with me whenever she wished.

When I went back in late September it was into a somewhat strange situation. Several of my close friends from my previous period three years earlier had been appointed as lecturers and fellows of various colleges. I was also surrounded by 18 year-old undergraduates. In St Catharine's there were eight medical students in my year. We all had the same director of studies and the same tutor. Our subject supervisors were however slightly different. Dr Comline having caused me the problems with the college at which I was going to study, then refused to teach me. My physiology supervisor was my very close friend and previous flatmate Dick Hardy (Dr Richard Hardy). By this stage he was married and had been elected a Fellow of Fitzwilliam College. My anatomy supervisor was Dr Michael Message with whom I had overlapped as a PhD student. My biochemistry supervisor was Dr Chris Thorne who was also my tutor.

Cambridge has a slightly unusual system of naming the posts that people may hold. A lecturer is a university appointment and is specific to a subject. The lecturer may or may not be a Fellow of a College. The Fellows are appointed by a College and may or may not teach within the College or the University. The majority of them are academic. There is nobody called a student. People studying are either undergraduates or postgraduates. Each undergraduate will have a supervisor in each subject that they are studying. The supervisor will meet his or her undergraduates in a group of one to four, and normally on a weekly basis during terms. Each undergraduate will have a more senior Director of Studies in their subject for advice on occasions, but they are not directly involved in teaching, and this person may be within or outside their own College. Each College will have between four and approximately eight tutors who are appointed to oversee the progress of the undergraduates that are allocated to them. This is normally on a term basis, but if there are problems, help or advice can happen very much more often. This can be of major advantage to any undergraduate in trouble, either academically or personally. Normally the appointment is within a range of subjects. For instance, my tutor, Dr Thorne, was a biochemist, and would have had within his care all of the biological scientists and the medical students and the veterinary students. Postgraduates have a research supervisor within their department and a postgraduate tutor within their College. Needless to say Oxford University has a different system which I will explain later.

Undergraduate teaching is done both within the University and within the College, and this is a major difference to most Universities. When term started all undergraduates had lectures, but the medical undergraduates were the only group that had six nine-o-clock lectures a week. We also had anatomical dissection and laboratory sessions in physiology and in biochemistry. We would all have been used to laboratories, but the dissection room was very different. The smell of the preserving fluid was very distinct and will never be forgotten by a medical student of those days for the rest of their lives. And as we went in, the sight of 80 dead bodies on tables, although each covered by a sheet, had an effect on us all. I, and I am sure many others, had never seen a dead body before. The effect on two of our group was such that they immediately left and changed the subject that they were to study. One of the two was the son of a famous orthopaedic surgeon whose textbook I used for years afterwards. I think that there was a chance that the lad had been pushed by his father, and was an unwilling medical student even before he started. The two hundred and forty of us were allocated, three or four to a body, and met the lecturers and demonstrators who were to teach us. The demonstrators were normally recently qualified doctors who were spending six months or a year preparing for the extremely difficult Primary examination for the Fellowship of the Royal College of Surgeons (Chapter 11). I am pleased to say that human dissection still carries on in Cambridge. Very many medical schools have now stopped it, and when I have been examining during the last few years, I have been upset by the lack of the knowledge of anatomy, not only in medical students but also in young surgeons.

During the first year I also added an extra subject of mathematics and statistics for medical students. In fact this turned out to be statistics and mathematics, and not having done any serious statistics before I found it hard work and spent very little time doing it as it was not a necessary qualification. The other problem that I had throughout that year was accepting biological mathematics. In biology 2 + 2 is roughly equal to 4; it may be a bit more or it may be a bit less. As a physical scientist 2 + 2 had always equalled 4, and in the laboratories I was always looking for a non-existent precise answer.

A normal undergraduate in Cambridge had to be in Cambridge for a full nine terms of eight weeks to enable them to be awarded a Cambridge degree. I had committed to return to Guildford to give my lectures in biochemical engineering on ten Fridays during that first year, but as I had previously done my 'terms' the requirement did not apply to me.

Towards the end of the summer term, Chris Thorne warned me that if I did not do some biochemistry revision I would do very badly in the examination. I did some revision, but not much, and very luckily part of the examination was a compulsory calculation. This was meant to take 40 minutes of the three-hour examination, and I was struggling to finish it in the time. It actually took me 45 minutes. I then wrote short notes on the other subjects, and much to the annoyance of Chris Thorne (who is still a friend), it turned out that I was the only person out of 300 people taking the examination that had got the calculation correct. Biochemistry was the only first-class pass of my Cambridge degree.

My social life during the year had gone through a major disaster. When I went back to Cambridge my engagement was going well, but my then fiancée Moira Megaw was having some recurrent psychological problems and was having discussions with a vicar as her adviser. The problems became larger, and after about four weeks of the first term our engagement broke up. For the rest of my two years in Cambridge there was no one else to whom I was particularly attracted and for the two May Balls that I attended, old girlfriends were invited. Very luckily sport helped me through this difficult time. I was playing five sports at College level, ice hockey at University and British Universities level, and sailing with the possibility of Olympic selection. These are discussed further in chapters 15 – 21. At the end of my first year, and I now no longer remember why, somebody had suggested that I should stand to be President of the Cambridge University Medical Society. Very unusual for a person only about to become a second year undergraduate. Surprisingly I was elected as Vice President.

By the end of my first year I was not particularly happy. My engagement had broken up, and I was still having some difficulty accepting the difference between the precise sciences of physics and of chemistry, and the imprecise science of biology.

I went home to stay with my mother for a few weeks before returning to Cambridge for the Long Vacation Term. As an engineering student I had had to spend three long vacation terms in industry. Several universities run extra courses in the summer for people who have failed the examinations, but I only know of Cambridge that had what was in effect an extra complete academic term. The purpose of the six weeks was an introduction to pharmacology with lectures and practicals. The subject had to be done at some time, and as I was doing a two-year short course using the vacation term meant that I would have finished my second MB examination with finals the next year, and not have to carry the pharmacology. It was certainly not hard work, and there was ample time for sport and social meetings. For a change cricket became my main sport. We played a team of the lecturers, and the University also ran a team with members from various colleges to play touring teams from around England and from overseas. I was selected for two of these, and one I remember particularly well. We were playing a team of colonial officers from around the world. A groundsman from one of the colleges had been a county spin bowler, and I will now admit that we put him in our team as a ringer. I was keeping wicket and had never kept at that sort of level of leg break bowler before. He indicated to me to stand up behind the wicket which I did. As he bowled, I could hear the fizzing of the ball which came down at about the same speed as a normal college fast bowler. It bounced outside the leg stump, spun viciously and hit me. The batsmen turned to me and said,

"I did not see that."

My reply was,

"Neither did I."

With the groundsman's help we won easily.

I did very little work on the pharmacology which, although well taught, was not very interesting, and at the exam of the end of the term, having done no work, I unfortunately failed by just one mark.

The last four weeks of that summer I returned to teaching at the Youth Hostels Association sailing centre at Maldon in Essex.

At the start of my second year I had committed myself to a variety of activities.

On a university level I had been elected Vice President of the Cambridge University Medical Society, and I was involved in both the University and British Universities ice hockey teams.

On a college level. although an undergraduate, I had been elected the President of the Middle Common Room (consisting of graduates), and that is where I met Brian Sweeney, who some years later was to have a major effect on the rest of my life by introducing me to my wife. I continued the discussion group of the younger fellows and the research students that I had started four years previously, and I was involved in badminton, squash, tennis, cricket and athletics, all at cuppers level (the intercollegiate competitions).

At least I had finished travelling to Guildford on some Fridays to give the biochemical engineering lectures, and having failed to get into the British Olympic team, had stopped competitive sailing.

The first thing that I had to do on returning at the beginning of term was to retake my pharmacology examination. I had done some work and I passed easily. The main subjects for the year were anatomy, especially neuroanatomy, physiology and pathology. My anatomy supervisor continued to be Dr Michael Message, my physiology supervisor changed to Dr Nankevill, and my pathology supervisor was Dr Kellaway. The medical undergraduates continued with six 9 o'clock lectures each week and we continued to work in the dissecting room with the dissection of the face and in the laboratories with neuroanatomy. We attended both the physiology and the pathology laboratories twice a week. There was one marvellous occasion in a pathology lecture which was being given by Dr Kendall Dixon, a fellow of King's College, who was known to be severely deaf. To reduce the chances of external noises upsetting his lecture he would always take his hearing aids out before starting. On that particular day he was giving the lecture about syphilis around the world. Unfortunately he had given exactly the same lecture the week before. There was considerable barracking which of course he could not hear. Eventually somebody got up and wrote on the board.

"This is last week's lecture."

"Oh," said Dr Dixon, and promptly gave the lecture that he should have been giving. The physiology and pathology lectures were excellent. Unfortunately one cannot say the same about many of the anatomy lectures with the exception of the embryology lectures by Dr Max Bull. He had a remarkable and unusual skill of being able to draw on the board, which was then the normal in lectures, with both hands at the same time. As many things in embryology are bilateral this was extremely useful, and as well as speeding up the lectures, made them much more comprehensible. The only other lectures in anatomy that I remember were on the human hand, which were given by Dr Malcolm Potts with appropriate and often amusing demonstrations. There were also occasional viva examinations in the anatomy dissection room during the year.

And that is the summary of my memories of the academic part of the second year course. One of the problems of the Cambridge lectures were that they were given in a generic form to cover all animals as well as humans. This was necessary because undergraduates other than medical ones attended the lectures. It did mean, however, that clinical aspects related to human beings were rarely mentioned. I only remember in one of the pathology lectures patients being brought into the lecture theatre to demonstrate neurological problems. Unfortunately one of the undergraduates watching the patients promptly fainted and had to be resuscitated by the lecturer.

During that year I was invited by my old friend Roger Tapp to a Fellows' Commemoration Dinner in Clare College. Apart from being an excellent and well watered dinner, I remember two things that happened at that dinner, the first was that I was sitting next to Sir Eric Ashby, a previous Master of Clare College, but then long retired. During our conversation he told me that when he had first been appointed as a Fellow, the College were expanding their accommodation for the undergraduates. He pointed out to the then Master that they were somewhat short of bathrooms. The Master replied,

"Why do they need baths – they are only here for eight weeks."

The second of the chance conversations from the dinner has had a lasting effect on my life. I was sitting next to Mr John Withycombe on my other side. He was one of the first urological surgeons in the country, and before we left he said to me that at any time that I wished to come in to Addenbrooke's Hospital, I could come and watch him operate. Luckily my memory was still working well, and the next day I went into the hospital to find Mr Withycombe. He looked at me somewhat puzzled, and I reminded him about his invitation of the preceding day at which an element of memory must have come over him, and he welcomed me. For the rest of that year I continued to attend his operating sessions on a regular basis, and at the end of the year I must have impressed him to some extent as he offered me his house job when I had qualified. A marvellous system now overtaken by political correctness.

Having finally finished with my engineering teaching I found the second year with no responsibilities very difficult. The Cambridge University Medical Society compensated to some extent for this difficulty. The President had asked me to do two things. Firstly to organise the lectures to be given by visiting speakers to all of the undergraduates who were members of the society. I decided to do this on the basis of a series of lectures looking to the future. The future of surgery would be by Prof Roy Calne, the future of medicine by Dr Geraint James, the future of embryology by Prof W J Hamilton and the future of biological science by Gordon Rattray Taylor, a well-known author. And then by chance the famous South African transplant surgeon Professor Christiaan Barnard announced that he was coming to Cambridge, and I persuaded him to give a lecture to the undergraduates. The second thing that the President asked me to do was to organise the blood donor week for the whole of the University. This was a very interesting challenge, and as always very few people were interested in giving blood. I arranged with a local brewery that, as a charitable donation, they would give a pint of beer to every donor, and a barrel of beer to the college who had given the largest donation on a proportional basis. There was no doubt whatsoever that this helped, and the week was the most successful on record. It was also the first time that I had actually donated blood as I felt I had had no option.

As a medical student in most universities one does the whole of the course in the same university. Only at St Andrews University in Scotland and in Cambridge did one have to change universities halfway. The reason for this at Cambridge was interesting, and could only really happen at somewhere as strange as Cambridge. In all other university medical schools, clinical lecturers are paid more than lecturers in other subjects. Cambridge had always believed that lecturers in all subjects were equal and had resisted this, and had accepted that they would therefore have a problem running a clinical medical school on those terms. We all therefore had to apply to do our clinical years elsewhere. I was strongly advised that if I wanted to be an NHS consultant in the future that I should apply to a London medical school. My anatomy supervisor Dr Michael Message suggested that Oxford would be more appropriate for me, and I still thank him very sincerely for his advice. I therefore applied to Oxford and was invited for an interview. It was a very different interview from those that my colleagues were receiving in London. We spent the whole day in Oxford, seeing a birth, a post-mortem and an operation, and having time to talk to the medical students who were there. At 5 o'clock we were interviewed, and I was offered a place. To cover the odds, I had also applied to University College Hospital, London and the following week went there for an interview. It was very different. I was shown into a large room with five or six elderly gentlemen making up the interview panel. The first question was,

"Did your father train here?" The answer was no. The second question was,

"Which members of your family did?" To which the answer was none.

The interview then went in fits and starts until somebody, having looked at my previous life, asked whether I thought that there was any future for computing in medicine. I made up some thoughts and told them, on no evidence, how important it was going to be. It turned out that the hospital had just bought a computer and did not know what to do with it. My input would therefore be useful. And finally one elderly gentleman, who had not previously spoken, asked me if I had applied anywhere else. I replied that I had applied to Oxford, to which he said that if University College offered me a place I would hopefully be coming here. I politely said that I thought that I would be going to Oxford. They must had been desperate for somebody to run their computer as they did still offer me a place. However, Oxford was very strongly my choice, and in retrospect it was very much the correct decision.

Finally that year we had the annual dinner of the Medical Society and I was sitting next to Dr Gordon Ostlere who was much better known as Richard Gordon, the author of very amusing medical fiction which included *Doctor in the House*. He had always been a hero of mine and I was looking forward enormously to the dinner, which turned out to be a major disappointment as I could get very little out of him during the whole evening.

Then came the examinations and award of my degree in the Senate House. I had compressed what is frequently a three year course into two. Apart from my unexpected success in the biochemistry examination, I had slipped by one mark into the class 2.2 level, or as it was known, a Desmond, after Archbishop Desmond Tutu.

A marvellous two years of Cambridge with all its attractions.

And then off to Africa.

FIVE

UNIVERSITY OF ZAMBIA

When I was finishing my preclinical two years at Cambridge, I knew that I would have some months to travel and ideally to do something useful. I therefore wrote to some six hospitals in Africa asking if they could use a medical student for three or four months. One of these places was a hospital in Zululand (Chapter 7), from which I had an answer saying that they would be delighted to have me when I was a clinical student, but as a preclinical student I would be of little use to them. I had no answer from four of the places, and then suddenly from out of the blue came a request for me to teach anatomy at the new university medical school in Zambia. (Photo 5.1).

Originally I had intended paying for myself to go to Africa, but Zambia not only offered to pay me, but also through a scholarship from the Anglo-American Mining Company said

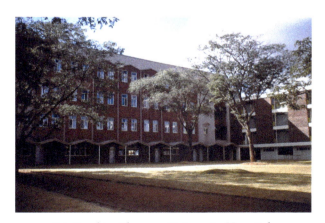

5.1 Zambia. The new University Hospital. This was opened after I had left. I taught anatomy and pathology to the first year medical students at the new medical school.

that they would pay my fare as well. And so in the June of 1969 I was appointed a Demonstrator in the University and set off for my first visit to Africa. The plane was an ancient 707 which had belonged to Italian Airways, and it was slightly off-putting that there was a notice saying that the Pope had travelled in the plane very many years earlier. At about 3 o'clock in the morning we arrived to refuel in French Equatorial Africa. This was my first experience of Africa, and I still remember the incredible humidity and temperature that hit me when the cabin door was opened. I also remember armed guards lining both sides of our walkway from the plane into the terminal, though who might have wanted to escape was not at all obvious. And then on to Lusaka where I was met and taken to the medical school. The medical school was some three or four miles away from the main University buildings and was situated adjacent to the main hospital of Lusaka, the capital city of Zambia.

I was introduced to Prof Miller and to the one other full-time member of the anatomy department staff, Dr Singh. The medical school was only in its first year since its foundation and consisted of about 24 students in the year. I had my accommodation arranged in a room in the medical school alongside the students who were nearly all resident. The students were a mixed band, mostly from Zambia, but there were three students who were South African coloured people, and one English lass whose parents were working in Zambia. There were also two other local lady students. The syllabus was discussed between the three of us, the Professor, Dr Singh and myself, and the human dissections and the lectures arranged.

Teaching in Zambia was very different from learning in Cambridge. Almost none of the students had had any books of their own, but they had an amazing ability to learn from what few books they had had available to them in school. Clearly their education up to then had totally depended on this amazing memory. And so the first week started with me giving some lectures, arranging some dissections, and getting to know the students. I also met and talked to the other members of staff teaching physiology and pathology. Amongst these was another student from Cambridge, Alan McGregor, who was there to teach physiology on the same basis that I had been appointed to teach anatomy. African students were incredibly respectful of their lecturers, much more so than I was used to in Cambridge, and it therefore took me some time to get to know them. It helped that two of the students were very good tennis players and with these I started to play tennis on the local courts. For the first time ever for me I had to use ball boys as this was a means of giving some money to local lads. The effect of this was that as soon as a point was decided the next ball was given to you – very exhausting, and especially at that altitude! I also, through some of the other lecturers in the medical school arranged a game of squash. This was also a nasty surprise, for at that time I was a very competent squash player having played at university level. I was upset to be beaten by somebody who was not nearly such a good squash player as myself, but he was used to playing at an altitude of some 4000 feet – the height above sea level of Lusaka. I would add that by the time I had got used to the altitude some two or three weeks later he rarely scored a point against me. After I had been there some days, I was invited to a party in the hospital and met an obstetrician/gynaecologist. He said that I would be welcome to join him in a clinic at any time, and as my anatomy teaching was by no means full-time, I did so the following day. He taught me how to examine a pregnant lady, to work out which way up was the baby, how to take a blood pressure, and, most importantly, how to fill up the relevant forms.

Having very much enjoy enjoyed my three hours in the obstetric clinic I went back the next week. The doctor running the clinic said that he was delighted to see me. His colleague who should have been in the next door room was ill, so would I please go next door and he would send me some patients. And so after two hours clinical experience I was examining patients and going through all the relevant questions on the form. One of these questions was 'Had anything strange happened to them since they were pregnant'. And the lady that I will never forget said that she had a lump in the back of her throat which had developed since she became pregnant. I looked in and there indeed was a lump on the side of the base of her tongue. I had no idea what it could be which was a little worrying and so I said that I would show this to my friend next door. I therefore got the obstetrician from next door to come and have a look. He also had no idea what it was, and therefore referred her to the ear, nose and throat surgeon. Some few days later he was a little upset to receive a message asking, 'why had he not recognised a lingual thyroid.' In fact this is a very unusual embryological variant. Our thyroid gland starts, when we are a few weeks old within the womb, from the back of our tongue and then migrates over the next few weeks down into the neck where it remains and functions for the rest of our lives. On occasions part of this track is not obliterated and one of the things that can happen in pregnancy is that a piece of the thyroid which had remained from where it started can expand, and this is what had happened to this lady. I will say that in the whole of my career I have only seen one other person with the condition.

The two of us demonstrators were looked after socially very well, both by our professors and by Dr Singh and his wife. We both bought bicycles, but the locals were not at all used to Europeans cycling around and we did indeed get some very strange looks as we cycled around the city and the surrounds. (Photo 5.2).

With my very respectful students I had no problems in the teaching, but did have to work very hard to keep up with their incredible memories. One thing that I did learn was their respect, which was almost total, of the written word. At one point I had said something, and one of the students pointed out that that was not what the book said. I therefore showed them the book that I was using and which was more up-to-date, and pointed out that the book they had was a little bit ancient. They were completely and utterly shattered by the fact that something written in a book could be wrong. We then had a long discussion about how knowledge does progress and that everything that is written in a book may or may not be correct. Clearly a concept that they had never considered.

Outside the department social life started slowly. There was a television in the students' mess, which was itself interesting in that often a film in different parts would be shown in the wrong order, and the advertisements might include a request to find a lost cat. Alan and I cycled around the town to see what was interesting, and we also at one point cycled up to the main university buildings about three miles distant. My professor was himself interested in birds and with my interest we would occasionally go birdwatching together. He would appear before lunch and ask what I was doing that afternoon, and if it could be arranged he drove us into the bush to do some birdwatching. He was not particularly knowledgeable, and when we saw something that he did not recognise

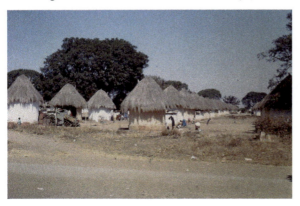

5.2 Zambia. A semi-official township just outside Lusaka. Whilst working at the university there was time to visit around the country.

he would describe it as an LBJ. At that time Lyndon Baines Johnson was the American President and it took me some time to work out that an LBJ describing a bird was a Little Brown Job and had nothing to do with the President. Prof Miller himself was a professor of anatomy at the University of California medical school and had volunteered to go to Zambia for three years to teach. His wife in the States was an attending anaesthesiologist (the equivalent of a British consultant) and it was interesting, when I got to know them better, to discuss the finances of American medicine. It turned out that in California his salary as a full-time and quite senior academic would only just pay for her medical malpractice insurance cover as an anaesthesiologist.

After about three or four weeks, the social life improved. I got to know some of the nurses, several of whom were European, and in particular British nurses, working out there for six months or a year. They were known locally as the 'sunshine sisters'. I also began to meet other members, particularly of the surgical staff, and those working in the accident department. 1969 was the time of the Biafran war in Nigeria and several of the junior surgeons and anaesthetists were Biafran. The chief surgeon in the hospital was a Scotsman, and the head of the accident department was an American. At this time the very few Zambian doctors that existed had almost all been trained in Russia, and were of a very variable, and often poor standard. In mitigation I would say that a Zambian going to Russia had to learn both Russian and Latin to be able to learn medicine and were at a major disadvantage. In the evenings I started attending the accident department regularly and was taught how to examine patients and how to sew up their wounds. These weeks were my first introduction to clinical medicine. I rapidly realised just how little I knew, not surprisingly, but it started me reading about the subject of medicine. If I am honest this was the first time in my life that I had really started working at the books. As I have said earlier, learning from books had always been easy for me, and I had never really needed to work hard to pass exams. Suddenly it became important that I knew what I was seeing and doing, and how to treat the various problems that were presenting in a casualty department. I became more and more involved in working in the hospital, not only in casualty but also assisting in the operating theatres.

Within the medical school I was mainly involved in teaching anatomy, and was then also asked to teach in the Department of Pathology. The other person with whom I had a considerable interface was Prof Maurice King who came to the medical school as a professor at the end of my first month. Prof King was a very famous professor of social medicine. He had been professor at the Makerere University Medical School in Uganda and had written several highly recognised textbooks on managing medical problems in Africa, particularly in the laboratory.

In Zambia in 1969 medicine was mainly provided by medical assistants working in clinics in the bush. These, nearly all male, would have had one or two years of training, and were at a lower level than a qualified nurse in Britain. Some of the bigger villages might also have a nurse, but there were virtually no doctors outside the major towns. One of Prof King's jobs was both to teach and to assess the medical assistants, and then to see how they were managing. On one occasion he invited me together with a European physiotherapist, and interestingly also a man from the Treasury in England who was visiting to see what was happening to the money that the English government was putting in to help medical care in Zambia. We got into Prof King's Land Rover and drove north out of Lusaka and after about an hour and a half of tarred road turned onto the bush tracks to visit three medical centres situated right in the middle of the forest. The local medical assistants were absolute experts at the ten common problems that they saw, and were able to diagnose, treat and prescribe for these ten conditions. If anything more complicated occurred in the clinics, or surgery was necessary, then the patients were transferred to the University Hospital in Lusaka. As it was getting dark and we were returning in the Land Rover the fan belt unfortunately broke. I asked Maurice where he kept his spare, at which he gave me a slightly unusual look, wondering what a spare fan belt might be doing in his Land Rover. Unfortunately our physiotherapist was not wearing tights – the standard replacement for a fan belt – and I therefore fixed the Land Rover by using Maurice's tie. This at least luckily lasted until we got back onto the tarred road by which time full night had descended – at which point it gave up. There were of course in those days no mobile phones and there was no way of contacting anybody in Lusaka some 40 or 50 miles away. We had been standing on the side of the road for a short time when a large lorry appeared. It was loaded with sacks of local maize and with a whole lot of people on top, clearly under the influence of alcohol, singing away happily. The driver went through his complete selection of odd fan belts that he had in his spare case, but unfortunately none of them fitted. Our visitor from the Treasury was therefore asked to go with the driver back into Lusaka. Maurice gave him the address of a friend who had a Land Rover, and he was to come back with the friend and a spare fan belt. Clearly this was a very memorable voyage for our civil servant. Some hours later he reappeared in the Land Rover of Maurice's friend with a fan belt. This I quickly fixed and we drove happily back to the medical school.

Very many years later I met this treasury person by complete chance at a dinner in a Cambridge college and somehow our joint visits to Zambia came into the conversation. It is always amazing how these things happen as neither of us recognised the other. He did say that his main memory of Zambia was the trip back to Lusaka with a lot of very drunken Africans happily singing away on top of the lorry. Maurice was clearly one of those brilliant academics, but really was not the most practical person you will ever come across – but I did make sure that there was always a spare fan belt in his Land Rover in an attempt to prevent future disasters, though whether he would be able to fix it I was doubtful.

There were three other major outside visits during my four months in Lusaka. The first was to visit Ndola – the main city of the copper belt in the North of the country where the Zambian flying doctor service was based. The flying doctor service was staffed by junior doctors coming out from Europe, and again mostly from Great Britain, and they flew with a nurse and a local medical assistant to the various clinics situated in the Bush. Their main role was to bring back people with serious injuries or medical conditions, or those needing surgery, but they would also do clinics in the various centres to which they were sent. These really were a complete waste of government money which would have been far better spent on other medical situations. In general these young doctors flying out had had no experience of African medicine, and little experience of recognising some of the tropical diseases and other problems that were locally common and well looked after by the medical assistants. The particular trip that I remember was a flight to a small landing strip on the Congolese border. I sat in on a clinic and began to talk to the locals through a translator. They had just trapped a small elephant in a drop pit and had slaughtered it and were drying out the meat on their very basic huts to make biltong. Elephants interestingly have very few hairs, but I did buy the hairs from the tail for about sixpence (2.5p) from which I made a small wrist band for myself. Elephant hair wrist bands were well known to bring good luck – and with my subsequent career it seems to have worked. They also organised for us a trip in very narrow dugout canoes across the river into the Congo (Photo 5.3). A short time walking around in the forest within the Congo followed. There were needless to say no border guards. We therefore could not

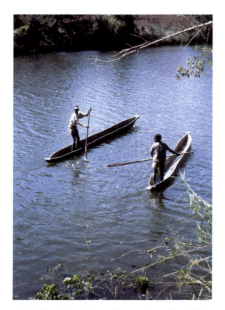

5.3 The Zambian Congo border. We flew there with the Zambian Flying Doctor Service and were paddled across in dugout canoes.

enter the country officially, and a Congo stamp is still not in my passport.

Our second trip was with Alan and the secretary to the Department of Anatomy, who was an Australian lass of about 30. She was rather large and owned a very small Fiat 500 car. We had a week off and organised ourselves to go south to Rhodesia. At that time Rhodesia was of course in the situation of UDI (Unilateral Declaration of Independence) with Ian Smith still controlling it. We had several interesting experiences on this trip. The first one was going down to the Victoria Falls and stopping on the bridge that joined Zambia to Rhodesia (now Zimbabwe). We were happily taking photographs there when the Zambian border guards and police arrived and accused us of spying. We pointed out that we actually had Zambian work permits in our passports and had been working in the University. Suddenly the whole attitude changed, and we were told that we were welcome to take as many photographs as we liked and go wherever we liked. They were delightful people and were clearly very happy then to see us knowing where we were working in Lusaka, and that we had no connections with Rhodesia (Photo 5.4).

That night we stayed in the famous hotel by the Victoria Falls on the Rhodesian side. The menu for dinner was given to us. There was a large choice of what we could have for every course. Being British, and even Australian, we selected one item for each course. We later found out that we could have had every single thing on the menu, and very soon staying in other hotels that is exactly what we did. We therefore ate very well throughout the whole of our ten day trip. Part of this trip was to the Wankie National Park. This was, in those days, an absolutely superb nature reserve. I understand now that tragically it has been over-hunted and over-poached, and it is no longer anything like the reserve as we had seen it. When there we had been warned about being careful and staying in our vehicles at all stages. A little later we were happily

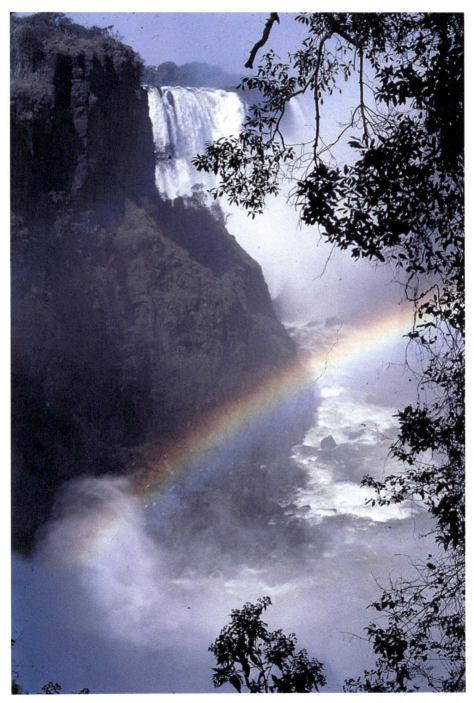

5.4 The Victoria Falls on our way to Rhodesia. That year there was the ideal flow of water. Very impressive but not too much to blanket the falls with spray.

photographing when we had the inevitable puncture. There were no other cars around, and we sat there wondering what to do. We eventually wound the windows down and clearly there were no animals to be seen. The real worries were both buffalo and male elephants, the latter particularly when separated from family parties. None were visible or audible and eventually I got out and changed the tyre. We drove about 50 yards around the corner and there was a very large male elephant happily munching at the vegetation.

Rhodesia has had an interesting selection of name changes. It started off as Southern Rhodesia, and when Northern Rhodesia became Zambia, Southern Rhodesia became Rhodesia. It is now Zimbabwe. One of the places that we did visit were the famous Zimbabwe ruins. These are a fascinating selection of stone buildings. It has never really been worked out who built them or when. But the famous Zimbabwean ruins are the origin of the present name of the country. At that stage although very much a colonial country, there was a general happiness and level of financial success which was different from, and a much greater happiness than in Zambia. My wife and I returned in 1974 as Government Medical Officers working in Marendellas. (Chapter 10).

Our third expedition away from Lusaka was to the Kafue National Park in the western part of Zambia. By this stage Alan and I had bought a wreck of a Morris Minor car between us. This car had a broken chassis and was just about usable within the city. A very kind 'sunshine sister' in the hospital, when we said we were taking this car to Kafue told us we were not taking that car and she would lend us her car instead. And so in her car the two of us drove west on a bush road. My first memory of driving along this road was to be happily driving on an almost empty road and suddenly would receive a vicious sting from a tsetse fly on any part of our body. Tsetse flies are extremely unpleasant. They are quite large – about the size of a wasp – but they silently land on clothes and actually sting through clothes. One therefore has no idea that they are around and there is no way of removing them before they sting. The sting itself is unpleasant, but may also carry the virus of the sleeping sickness disease. Luckily with the many times we were stung, neither of us caught sleeping sickness, which in those days was probably incurable. When we arrived in The Kafue Reserve we were the only visitors and the local reserve manager, a Zambian white gentleman was delighted to see us. He gave us very special and very memorable guided tours of the reserve with his incredible local knowledge. We spent three happy days doing this before driving back to Lusaka.

And so the anatomy and pathology teaching continued, and my increasing attendance and work within the hospital, and particularly in the accident department, increased. There was a desperate shortage of doctors and there were of course no medical students there as the medical students had not yet started the clinical parts of their training as it was only the first year since the foundation of the medical school. Anything I could do was therefore welcome. One always remembers the odd patient and, the odd situation. Two I remember well. The first was a patient that came in with very high blood pressure, and obviously unwell. He was a young man, and the story was that he had been bitten by a spider. There is in that part of Africa a dangerous spider – the button spider – related to the black widow spider of the West Indies, which can itself be fatal, but is rarely so. What was interesting about this patient was that the marks of the spider bite on his leg were some 3 cm in diameter. I know of no spider other than a tarantula which is anywhere near that size, and on questioning him about the size of the spider it turned out that it was about 7 mm long. How a spider 7 mm long could cause scarring about 3 cm across was not very clear until the sister in the department, who was a local lady , said,

"Oh, he's been to the witchdoctor first."

The witchdoctor had obviously scarified the area to make it bleed and to try and relieve the effect of the poison. His high blood pressure was treated, the wound covered and home he went rejoicing. The second patient I remember was a gentleman who was bought in unconscious by two policemen. He had a low pulse rate, a low blood pressure and very slight movement on a painful stimulus. By this stage I had done a lot of reading, I went through every cause of unconsciousness I could recall and none of them fitted. Again the local sister came to the rescue when she took one look at this gentleman said,

"Oh, he has been bewitched" I asked, totally astounded.

"What do you do with people who have been bewitched?"

She took some gauze, put it across his mouth and nose and poured on liquid ammonia so that he was breathing extremely strong ammonia, but only for about a minute – at which stage he had suddenly become conscious and was howling round the department with the two policemen trying to catch him. They eventually caught him and bought him back to the examination couch, at which stage the sister wagged a large finger under his nose and said to him,

"White man's medicine is stronger than black man's medicine." I thought this was a little strong, but she said afterwards that had she not done that he would have gone out and could have died.

As I said earlier the shortage of doctors in the country was considerably helped by the presence of several Biafran doctors. They were in general very capable and very pleasant doctors who taught me a lot and were very happy to have me along at any time. As the weeks progressed I spent more and more time working in the casualty department and at the end of my four months in Zambia as there was nobody else, I was left in charge of the casualty department every night for a week in the main hospital of the capital city of the country. Certainly a challenge for a preclinical student, and before I had even started working on the wards in England.

What was my overall opinion of the four months in Zambia? It was certainly an interesting country having been independent only since 1964. The President, Kenneth Kaunda, had been without doubt an excellent choice of President. His father was a minister in the Church of Scotland, and interestingly the President himself was not from a family occurring in any of the 10 tribes that live in Zambia. He was actually of Malawian origin and therefore acceptable to everybody in Zambia. The vice president was a different proposition. He was a member of the Bemba tribe, which was based in the copper belt to the north of Zambia. He had been quoted at one point as saying that 'the only good white man was a dead man'. He in fact was demoted only two years after I left the country.

As I said there were ten tribes in the country (and all 10 tribes were represented in the capital Lusaka,) and this meant that translating was often difficult as many patients spoke little or no English. One had to find a member of staff who both spoke the tribal language and English fluently enough to translate medical problems. All of the medical students spoke English extremely well, and on brief meetings with students in other subjects, again their English was normally very good. I had no problems of any kind socially with any of the students, but those reading politics certainly found it more difficult to accept the fact that I was a foreign overseas lecturer.

The shops were often short of common necessities such as toothpaste, but in general this did not affect my normal life. The television was interesting (but at this time there was no television at all available in South Africa). Certainly the knowledge of the outside world was often somewhat missing. I well remember reading a letter in the Times of Zambia from a senior policeman. He said that he had watched the moon the whole of the night before and he did not see anybody land on it and he did not believe the Americans. This was actually the night on which the first rocket from the United States landed on the moon and which had been pre-advertised.

There were problems that were occurring throughout the country. I am sure that corruption was common in the country, but it really did not affect us in any obvious way. In fact the opposite almost happened. I had been driving our wreck of a car down the main road into the centre of Lusaka when I was radared. It was almost inconceivable that the police in Zambia had a radar machine, but that in fact was the case. Being a good boy, I paid my 10 kwatcha fine. However a few days later in the casualty department I was complaining to a senior policeman that I had been caught in their one radar trap and paid my fine. His immediate comment was,

"You did not pay the fine, did you?"

I explained that I had indeed done so. He said,

"Next time you get caught, don't pay the fine, come and see me and I will make sure it is cancelled."

At one time the wages of agricultural workers were doubled by the Government, but the farmers were not allowed to increase the price of their products. This of course led to a major problem, and what happened with some farmers was that they did not plant any crops that year. One other problem which took me some time to discover was that about one third of the medical students that I was teaching had very little interest in medicine, but needed the name Doctor in front of their names so that they could be elected as politicians.

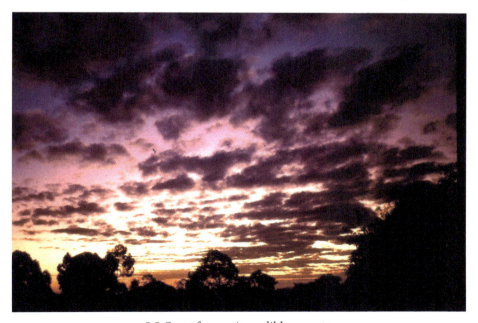

5.5 One of many incredible sunsets.

It was well known that everybody wished to become a Member of Parliament so they could acquire the three M's – Money, Mercedes and Mistresses.

Overall, my visit was absolutely marvellous. It was a beautiful country with amazing sunsets (Photo 5.5). I learned a lot, I realised how little I knew in the way of medicine, and the stress of being left in charge of the casualty department for every night for a week certainly made me work much harder both then, and on my return to England.

I regret that I have not had a chance to return to Zambia, but have at least visited many other countries in Southern Africa since my return. Who knows – one day.

SIX

UNIVERSITY OF OXFORD

Having returned from Africa I spent a couple of days with my mother and then having packed up my car drove to a completely new life based on the Radcliffe Infirmary in Oxford. I was a reformed character and actually working at the books for almost the first time in my life. The medical school then was in Osler House which was based just to the north of the main infirmary, with the famous Tower of the Winds in its grounds (Photos 6.1, 6.2 and 6.3). Osler House was the centre for all of the medical students, and the teaching was done in various parts of the various hospitals. Very luckily on the notice board was the offer of a house sharing with three other medics in their second and third years. I went to look at No 11, Warnborough Road about half a mile north of Osler House. It was a large basement room, and although a little damp was perfect. I moved in.

North Oxford has been recommended as the best suburb in England in which to live. It has an interesting history. One

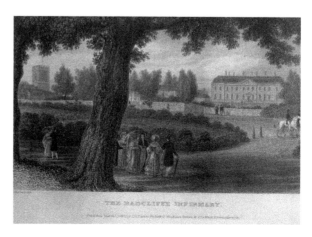

6.1 The Radcliffe Infirmary, Oxford in 1834

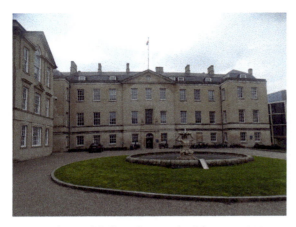

6.2 The Radcliffe Infirmary building in 2022. This is now the Blavatnik School of Government.

story is that it was built in the 1870s after the Oxford and Cambridge Act of 1877 had allowed dons to be married and to live in Oxford. Their wives moved from London, or anywhere else where they had been living unrecognised. If this is true, there must have been a lot of them as North Oxford has a large number of houses of the same vintage. Most of the houses are red brick, tall and elegant in wide roads, of which Warnborough Road, which runs parallel to Banbury Road between Leckford and Farndon Roads, is one.

I was settling in happily when a few weeks later I had a telephone call to say that my mother had been admitted to Whipp's Cross Hospital the previous night and had died overnight. She had been ill on and off for years, caused by her smoking, but although expected, it was still a severe shock, and particularly as I had nobody close to me to share it with. I let Mr Tidy, the medical school secretary know and drove to Whipps Cross Hospital. I collected the death certificate and her belongings and then drove home to work out what next to do. Our next door neighbour but two was a young solicitor who was incredibly helpful. He organised the cremation, the will and probate, and the sale of the little bungalow which, apart from a few hundred pounds, was the main part of my inheritance. Most of this he did after I had returned to Oxford. There was a small family cremation in the City of London Crematorium where her ashes remain. The bungalow sold for £9,000 and after my thanks to the solicitor, settling my debts and saying goodbye to my old neighbours I collected some items from the house, but even left my old motor bike behind, and returned to Oxford. Having only just arrived in Oxford and just started making friends I was more alone than ever.

Over the next few weeks I started looking for a house to buy, and by complete chance found No 4, Warnborough Road for £8,500. Knowing the prices of the two houses now, the Oxford house was surprisingly cheap. I moved in, furnished it from newspaper adverts and rented out some of the rooms.

Whilst all this was happening I also had to find time to be a medical student. As might be expected of Oxford there was an unusual system for admission of the clinical medical students. There were two intakes each year which were six months apart. The October intake was mainly from Cambridge graduates who had already passed their pharmacology and pathology examinations. Six months later the Oxford intake was formally admitted as they had spent the previous six months doing their pathology and pharmacology. There were 80 Oxford pre-clinical undergraduates, of whom 25 remained in Oxford and the rest mainly went to London hospitals. My intake was 26 students, 20 of whom came from Cambridge, one from London, one from Swansea after completing his PhD, and the other four from Oxford after they had finished their research degrees. Interestingly of the 26 of us, as well as the higher medical degrees five had degrees in other subjects. For a change I was not the oldest of the group, a distinction held by Myra who had previously been an English teacher.

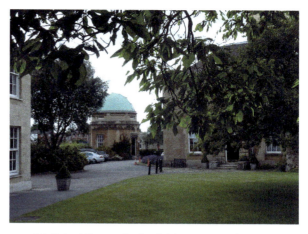

6.3 Osler House, Oxford. The centre where the medical students could meet, eat and drink. There were tennis and squash courts in the grounds.

The start for the new students was a six-week introduction to clinical medicine. This was a series of talks and demonstrations from a variety of lecturers telling us how firstly to examine patients, and secondly how to write the relevant notes required. As a medical student one then rotated through various firms. A firm consisted of all the people from consultant(s) down to the medical students in each specialty who worked together for a period of time. We were allocated to one of these firms in rotation. My first firm was general surgery with Mr Till and Mr Webster.

There were some very interesting consultants in Oxford, and few more interesting than Mr Tim Till. He was on the Council of the Royal College of

Surgeons, and also an examiner for the College. But as well as this he was Master of the local Foxhounds, and more importantly for us both an excellent surgeon and an excellent teacher. Mr Webster was based at the Churchill Hospital, some four miles away, and during our eight weeks of general surgery we had virtually no contact with him.

The sister on Mr Till's ward was Sister Wellington, unfortunately known as 'The Boot'. In the 1960s ward sisters had an enormous amount of power. Certainly getting to know them made life an awful lot easier, particularly for medical students who in the opinion of sisters were there just to bother their patients. I had an early set to with 'The Boot'. I had been sent to clerk one of the patients, and the notes were not in the usual place. I discovered that sister was having a meeting with nurses in her office and the notes were with her. I therefore knocked politely on the door and asked if I could have the notes.

"How do you know I have got the notes?" was her instant reply.

"I have been told that you have them." and the notes were given to me, but not with any good grace. Over the next few months and years I got to know Sister Wellington quite well and among the medical students I became a very rare friend of hers. A very lonely lady with few friends.

It is interesting how one remembers the sisters on the wards. They were often known, not by their own name, but by the name of the ward. One of the most famous of all was Sister Richard Lower (I never did discover her proper name). She was in her early 60s and close to retirement and was certainly well-recognised as a dragon whose care and comfort of the patients was by far the most important thing in her life. There were some marvellous stories about Sister Richard Lower. In the year above me there was a medical student some 10 years older than me. He was set up by his fellow students to do a ward round as Prof Smith, a famous professor from London. He was an excellent actor and I understand that the ward round was hilarious, and Sister Richard Lower did not at the time discover that she was being taken for a major ride. My first encounter with her was when one of Mr Till's patients was on her ward, and I had been sent to clerk him. In those days one politely asked the sister if one could examine patients, and her instant response was,

"Who are you?" I said I was,

"Roberts from Mr Till's firm",

"Are you the new registrar?"

"No" I replied, "I am the new medical student."

Older age had some major benefits. She was totally nonplussed with this, but having made an error allowed me on the ward without the usual problems she created. From then on, embarrassed by, and compensating for her bad mistake, we got on well. After I qualified Sister Richard Lower was compulsorily retired because of her age. It then turned out she had had a massive breast cancer which was ulcerated and pouring pus. She had done nothing about this as it would have taken her away from the care of her patients to have major surgery, or even worse, to be made to retire. A truly marvellous lady.

Another sister I knew was Sister Chris Harrison. She was of a similar age to me and came from the next door village to my own at home. I was on my first surgical firm at the time and one day was having tea with her in her office. One of the nurses came into the office in a panic to say Mr X was bleeding badly following an operation that day. We both rushed onto the ward and indeed Mr X was rapidly exsanguinating from his right groin where an operation had been carried out on his femoral artery. I immediately applied some pressure to reduce bleeding, and then handing this over to somebody, put an intravenous cannula into his arm to replace the blood that he was rapidly losing. This was the first ever intravenous cannula that I had inserted. I was thanked by Mr Gough, the surgeon whose patient it was when he arrived, and I later heard that Mr Till, in the consultant's mess was taking the mickey out of Mr Gough. saying that he understood that one of his first-year students had had to do the operation for him.

Other sisters that I remember well were in the neurosurgery unit. Sister Cambridge was in charge of the operating theatre, and was an incredibly helpful lady on many occasions when I was operating there later in my career. However on the ward was Sister Nuffield – again named after her ward. I arrived there as a student locum and introduced myself. She said hello and then looked at a desperately ill patient who was clearly dying in a bed near the sister's station. She asked me what I thought he wanted for his lunch. I did not understand the request at all as he was clearly totally incapable of eating anything. I apologised and said that I did not understand what she meant. She then looked straight at me and said,

"What do you think he wants for his lunch?"

For all the time that I was working on that ward I never bought myself a meal in the canteen.

After that short digression returning to my first three months. There was an open invitation for medical students to visit the accident and emergency department any evening or weekend if they wished to do so. After my experience in Zambia within a few weeks I was a regular attender in the Department. It was very different to Lusaka as there was an experienced team looking after the patients. The Oxford Accident Service was in the old Radcliffe Infirmary, and it was unusual in that the junior doctors working there looked after patients who had had accidents, and only in the emergency situation looked after those who were medically ill. These were kept alive until the junior doctors from the medical teams arrived, when they looked after them in an area away from the main Accident Department. There was also a rule that if the patient lived locally. they would only be seen if it was within 24 hours of the accident. Obviously if they were seriously ill they were looked after, but those with minor accidents outside this time limit were told to see their GP. The usual argument was that their GP was too busy, in which case the Department would phone the GP surgery and make the appointment for them. The vast majority of the local GPs were in total support of the arrangement which worked extremely well.

And so I would start seeing the simple patients in the Accident Service, suturing the wounds that weren't on the face, arranging x-rays and writing up the notes and putting on plasters of Paris. I spent several hours nearly every weekend working there and within a few weeks was doing more and more complicated procedures. Then came my first big chance. In those days, and tragically they no longer occur, when a junior doctor was on leave, with the agreement of the consultant a student would stand in for them. These were known as student locums. The student was clearly on trial and closely supervised. Legally, with the agreement of the consultant, they could do anything except sign for dangerous drugs or certify death. These student locums were normally in the third clinical year of one's training. It was astonishing that after I had only been there for about four months I was offered my first student locum in the Accident Service for, if I remember correctly, four days. I had to ask Mr Till for the time off from his firm. He looked at me in total astonishment and said that if they thought I could do it, I could have the time off. The locum included a room in the hospital and free food, but in the early days was unpaid. Knowing my inexperience, I had excellent backup from the junior doctors who were there. I remember needing to take some blood from a patient and failing to do so. An alternative method of taking blood when normal veins were not obvious was to take it from the femoral vein in the groin. This I had not done and very helpfully along came a junior pathology doctor to show me how to do it. That was typical of my many times as a locum.

Lectures were not a major part of the teaching. Every weekday evening there was a lecture at 6 o'clock and these were organised on a two year rotation. This allowed for periods when every student was away from the hospital or was tied up in the operating theatre or on the wards. The only lectures that were compulsory, and I understand a legal requirement, were the forensic pathology lectures. For some reason forensic pathologists are often well recognised as very amusing lecturers so one happily attended. The Oxford forensic pathology lectures (murders and major accidents etc.), were given by Prof Keith Simpson. I always remember his introduction.

"If you wish to buy a book on the subject, there are several available, but humility precludes me from recommending the best."

In my last days at Cambridge I went out with a fellow medical student Elspeth McAdam. She moved to the Middlesex Hospital for her clinical years and one time I went to London and went with her to one of her lectures which were much more part of her course then were ours. Although I should not base my judgement on one lecture, the level at which that lecture was delivered was way below that of the Oxford lectures. I realised again that I had made the right decision for my clinical years.

Back to Mr Till's team for the remainder of the two months. It was normal in those days for consultants to invite their junior doctors and four students for a meal or social occasion. We drove out to his house for a drinks party. One of his house surgeons at the time was Dr Christine Lee. She was very happily drinking away when Mrs Till came over and said to her that she was very sorry that she had to leave. Christine had had no intention of leaving, but did take what was a rather broad hint. Some months later there was the most marvellous story about Mr Till. I said earlier that he was the master of the local foxhounds and he appeared in the Accident Service in full hunting pink. Unfortunately the junior doctor that saw him had not trained at Oxford. Mr Till told him that he had injured his thumb. The junior doctor then came out of the small cubicle and said in a rather loud voice that a local country bumpkin had fallen off his horse and damaged his thumb. The doctor was then told that he had just seen the senior surgeon of the hospital and that he had better get back in and sort it all out rather quickly. When one got to know Mr Till one would have realised that he would have very much enjoyed the joke.

After two months on a surgical firm I then transferred to the medical firm of Dr Badenoch and Dr Hockaday. Dr Badenoch, an old style physician, was a delightful and very wise man who was later knighted for his services to medicine. Dr Hockaday was much younger and a good teacher but certainly did not stand idiots well. He was a good squash player and when he discovered that I had played at a good level asked me for a game. The only problem with Dr Hockaday, both medically and whilst playing squash, was that he would not give up. At one point I had him running from side to side of the court behind me until he was totally exhausted. He didn't ask me to play squash again. There was another social occasion when Dr Badenoch invited the students to his house for dinner. One of the students was a lady, Carol Barton, who was somewhat surprised that after the dessert course Mrs Badenoch invited her to powder her nose. In those days ladies leaving the men to their port was becoming extremely uncommon – except in the Badenoch house. The two months of medicine passed very well with me still working in the Accident Service at the weekends.

We were then allocated in small groups of four to ten to spend time in the various other departments both in the Radcliffe infirmary, and also in the specialist hospitals around Oxford.

Ophthalmology was done in the eye hospital which was in the grounds of the Radcliffe Infirmary but separated from it. There we were taught how to examine eyes, and also to test eyes and determine the strength of spectacles if they were needed.

Ear nose and throat, or otorhinolaryngology was done in the Radcliffe Infirmary at the same time as we were doing the eye work. Although I did not meet him then it was well known that an excellent retired ENT surgeon was still coming back to cover the colleagues in post when they were on holidays. He was 78 at the time, and had been made to retire at the age of 65, as was normal in those days.

The anaesthetics was much more interesting. It was a subject in which one could start to do something rather than just watch. One of the older consultants as well as teaching us about modern anaesthesia also showed us some of the old methods, in particular putting a gauze over the nose and mouth and pouring on the anaesthetic fluid. He also showed us the use of the EMO machine. EMO stood for East Mitchell Oxford and had been devised at the Radcliffe Infirmary by Mr East, the anaesthetic technician, and Dr Mitchell, the consultant, as a safe way of giving ether anaesthetics. When I was later working in Lesotho it was the standard machine, and I felt much happier having used it before. One day I went to assist an anaesthetist with an ENT operating list. I did much of the anaesthetic for him and when I appeared the following week, he said how delighted he was to see me as his registrar, who should have been in the next-door operating theatre, was ill. He therefore sent me next door to give the anaesthetics for a full operating list. My experience in Zambia had been of great value.

The psychiatry was in two different hospitals. The Littlemore hospital used drugs extensively in the treatment of their patients. The Warneford hospital treated patients by talking to them with very little use of drugs. My group was attached to the Warneford hospital where we were allocated two patients at the beginning. One of these was a long term patient, and the other an acute patient who had been admitted within the past few days. There was one well known long term patient who was certain that he was King Edward IX, and would talk to us about his family history. He had been a scholar as an undergraduate in one of the Oxford colleges and was extremely intelligent. Apparently during the Second World War he had learned Japanese so that he could join in the discussions over the peace process. A considerable number of undergraduates had psychiatric problems during their time at Oxford. The Warneford hospital always boasted that they had a higher percentage of first-class degrees from the undergraduates who were inpatients taking their final examinations than any other college. Towards the end of our eight week attachment we were given an examination and put in a room with a camera, a microphone and a patient. I was allocated a young girl who came into the room with her doll and then would not say a word. It is remarkably difficult to do a psychiatric examination in that situation. I eventually started talking to her doll and had a response from the young girl. Afterwards I was congratulated by the consultant for having managed to get anything out of her at all.

I have found throughout the whole of my career that psychiatrists are unusual. The consultants at the Warneford were very impressed when we would drop in to see our old long-term patient weeks and months later. I really do not think that it ever dawned on them that the reason was the food at lunchtime was both much better and much cheaper.

Psychiatry was certainly very different. There were three of us in my group who wanted to be surgeons. Peter Teddy, Terry Duffy, and myself. We had noticed that teaching psychiatry was very different to surgery. In those days, and perhaps unfortunately not now, if you said something stupid to a consultant surgeon he would not be very polite. If you said something stupid to a psychiatrist they would always say,

"Yes you might have a point but don't you think it could be…..?" The three of us tried very hard to get a psychiatrist to tell us we were idiots but failed miserably. I think that we all got a grade C for our psychiatric attachments.

The next attachment was to the Churchill Hospital to study plastic surgery, dermatology and radiotherapy for three weeks. This was my first introduction to plastic surgery which I found extremely interesting. At the end of my three weeks Mr Tom Patterson. the senior consultant. asked me to do a week as a student locum. Not a difficult decision, and I enjoyed it enormously. Clearly I must have been satisfactory as at the end of my locum he offered me a six month SHO appointment in the future.

The Oxford medical school had the lowest proportion of its graduates going into general practice of any medical school in the country. We did however all spend two weeks in a general practice to receive an understanding of the system. I organised my own two weeks; with a week in a town practice in Cambridge with Dr Anderson and a week in a country practice in Clifton Hampden in Oxfordshire. Dr Anderson I knew through sailing, and Dr Wilfrid Dickson I had met skiing. Certainly those two weeks were interesting, but did not attract me to general practice for a career. I understand that medical students now spend three months of their training in general practice, and they are now short of GPs, which was not the case in the 1970s.

We all spent six months doing clinical pathology in the laboratories and the post mortem room. Working down the microscope could often be a major challenge and sometimes interesting. Three of the twenty six of us finished up as consultant pathologists which must say something about both the teaching and the interest of the subject.

Geriatrics was an interesting six weeks. On our first introduction to the consultant, Dr Wollner, he told us that if we could not find six diagnoses for every one of the patients there was something wrong with us and not with the patient. It was a good challenge for the future. When I had been on the Accident Service, one of the jobs was to look after the ladies' trauma ward in which were a large number of elderly, or very elderly ladies, with fractured necks of femur. The experience gained during my geriatric attachment proved to be useful.

Combined neurosurgery and neurology were a short attachment. Having been involved in the care of head injuries doing my Accident Service student locums the more interesting part of this attachment was the neurosurgery. The Oxford Department of neurosurgery was world famous. The neurosurgeons were Mr Joe Pennybacker and Mr John Potter. When the American President John F Kennedy was shot, Mr Pennybacker was put into an American plane to fly to Texas to assist with his surgery. Apparently on the news of the president's death half way across the Atlantic it turned round and brought him back to Oxford. Mr Potter was the surgeon responsible for the introduction of compulsory helmets for all motorcyclists. His room was decorated with helmets showing the severity of the damage to them. There were two major advances in neurosurgery happening at this time. Firstly the CT scanner was invented, and secondly the Glasgow coma scale was being introduced to measure the severity of reduction in consciousness. Before the CT scanner was available the neurological examination of the patient and specialised arterial x-rays were critical in making an accurate diagnosis.

At the end of the attachment I was asked to do a student locum for head injury care as the full-time registrar was Mr Mohan was going on holiday for a week. I was therefore in a somewhat embarrassing situation that I was a student locum registrar with a fully registered senior house officer beneath me. Having done no neurosurgery before he was happy with the situation which was extremely helpful as it was the first week of the autumn term and we had nearly 50 undergraduates with head injuries from playing rugby. Luckily none of these were major and did not need surgery. I discovered afterwards that Mr Potter who was the head injury consultant had not realised that I was still a student and had thought that I was qualified and registered. He later gave me an excellent reference for a future job.

Then came orthopaedics at the Nuffield Orthopaedic Centre (NOC), some two miles away from the Radcliffe Infirmary. It was known amongst the students as the knocking shop. I cannot imagine why, but there were some attractive nurses! This hospital only dealt with cold orthopaedics as any accidents requiring orthopaedic input were treated at the Radcliffe. The Professor of Orthopaedics was Prof Robert Duthie who was known to be a martinet, not only to the students but even to his fellow consultants. Saturday morning at 9 o'clock was the main teaching session and he would be outside the door ticking everybody off from his list as they arrived, including his colleagues. Early in the eight weeks the students in my group had an examination from Prof. One of the ladies in my group was reduced to tears which we discovered afterwards was not uncommon when he was examining. When he came to me, he gave me a skull x-ray to diagnose. The diagnosis of multiple myeloma, a bone cancer, was particularly easy as I had recently done a medical prize essay on the subject. Having my fellow student upset I was not in a good mood, and made it very clear that I knew more about the subject than he did. Afterwards I was called into his room and thought that I was in serious trouble. In fact he congratulated me, offered me a research topic and a six months SHO appointment at any time in the future if I wished to have it. A definite case where it paid to fight back. Some seven or eight years later he was visiting the new Professor of Orthopaedics at Leeds University who had been one of his juniors. At that time I was the senior registrar in plastic surgery. We met, and he turned to me and said,

"You should have done orthopaedics." At least I could answer that hand surgery was to be a major part of my future career.

As well as the orthopaedic attachment we also had two months of working in the accident service. By this stage I had done several student locums and was let off four weeks of this attachment which I added to my elective time in South Africa.

The final specialty was obstetrics and gynaecology. I was allocated to the firm of Mr Arthur Williams. The firm was made up of the one consultant, a senior registrar Mr Alan Vass, a registrar and two house officers. Neither Alan Vass or I got on well with Mr Williams. As Alan had the job of organising the operating lists he would give the registrar, whom neither of us liked, to Mr Williams and Alan and I would operate on the second list. One of the problems was that whilst on the firm we were required to deliver ten babies. It was always difficult to beat the nurses and student midwives to each delivery. For some unknown reason the supervising midwives appeared to favour their student colleagues.

The last four months before the revision course were divided between general surgery and general medicine. My general surgery was with the Professorial team under Prof Allison. The story was that some years before whilst having an operation on himself he had had a cardiac arrest and although surviving, his mental state was not what it had been. He had been known to be one of the most brilliant academic surgeons in Britain. Unfortunately he did not retire, but neither did he operate again, and he ran his department from a distance. The consultant surgeons that I worked with most during these two months were Mr Lee and Mr Gunning. The senior registrar was Miss Tessa Morrell, at a time when lady general surgeons were extremely rare. To compete she knew that she had to be extremely aggressive and working with her was not easy. It was a less satisfactory time than the eight weeks that I had spent with Mr Till.

My last two months were spent with the medical firm of Doctors Grant Lee and John Ledingham. They were a complete contrast to each other. Dr

Lee was difficult, and Dr Ledingham absolutely delightful, both to us and to his patients. He also edited the Oxford Textbook of Medicine which is now a standard work. During this time I did a one week student locum in medicine for the Badenoch and Hockaday firm. It was an interesting time as there was a major flu epidemic in the country with a large number of nurses ill. My fellow medical students were recruited onto the wards to help with the nursing, and by complete chance I was in charge of them all.

In my three years I spent a total of between 12 and 14 weeks doing student locums. They were incredibly useful to add to the experience of being a medical student. In my first year they were completely unpaid but by the third year we were paid at the same rate as a hospital porter, and that also helped. And now they do not exist!

During my third and final year, and I still do not know how, I was asked to tutor anatomy for the medical students in St Edmund Hall, one of the Oxford colleges. To avoid confusion, tutoring in Oxford is the same thing as supervising in Cambridge, and in no way was I in charge of these undergraduates. Tutoring was very different to my lecturing in the University of Zambia and in many ways more enjoyable because of the small number in each group.

Having reached nearly the end of this chapter I realise how little I have written except about work. Although I was working very hard for these three years it was not exclusive to my life. I was certainly involved in sport both in Worcester College (Photo 6.4) with tennis, badminton and squash, in the University with badminton and ice hockey, and in the British universities team with ice hockey. I collected my half blue in ice hockey in my first year and my British universities colours that same winter. I organised skiing parties in both Easter vacations, and was also selected for the British Ski Club representatives' course in Davos in the second winter (1971). I was not involved in any other university clubs, but did dine regularly in college with the Middle Common Room.

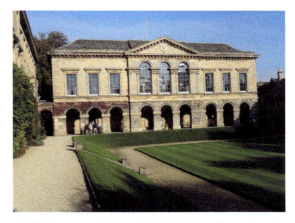

6.4 Worcester College, Oxford. My college when I was a clinical medical student at Oxford.

How it happened I do not remember but I was asked to be the marketing manager for the Oxford University Medical School Journal. This had been successful in the past, but was going through a somewhat lax period. When the new Journal was published. I took some to Blackwell's, the famous bookshop in Oxford. I approached the salesperson in charge of the medical section and asked him whether he could sell them for us. He suggested I went to talk to somebody on the top floor of the shop and directed me to see him. I knocked on the door and found a very elderly gentleman sitting behind a desk. I asked him whether it would be possible for the shop to sell them, and how much they would want to do so. We had a short talk and he then told me to go back to the medical section and Blackwell's would sell them for us and not charge. I asked the salesperson who I had been talking to, and to my amazement was told that it was Sir Basil Blackwell, the founder and owner of the shop. I worked out that he was 83 years old, and I have since discovered that he continued to work in the shop for a further five years to make 60 in total. An amazing man and an amazing shop.

My interest in young ladies returned during the three years and I had three or four fairly serious girlfriends. Unfortunately these were either overseas or in London at the time, which made life somewhat more difficult. In the August of my second year life changed for good, in both meanings of the word. A friend of mine from Cambridge, Brian Sweeney, had suggested to an ex-girlfriend of his, Vivian Onians, that I might have accommodation available for her in Oxford where she was going to continue her general practice training. In August she knocked on my door in Warnborough Road and we talked for some time. I then left a note on her car suggesting a game of mixed doubles squash with two other friends of mine. That was the start of our relationship although it turned out that she had already found accommodation but after a few weeks she moved in with me when I returned from Michigan – and she was not even charged. We became engaged at one minute past midnight on January 1, 1972 when we were visiting the Spurway family in Glasgow. Our original plan was to get married as soon as I had qualified, but we decided that finals and planning a wedding together might be difficult. We therefore moved the date forward to March 24 and had a very small wedding in the Cambridge registry office, followed by tea or coffee in the garden of Vivian's parents in Cambridge. We then joined the ski party that I had already arranged before I met Vivian. This was in Crans Montana and was our honeymoon. There was one double bed in the chalet and very kindly we were allowed the use of it.

Three months later after my finals, and getting to know many of each other's friends, we had a large dinner dance in the Graduate Society Centre beside the River Cam in Cambridge.

FINAL EXAMINATIONS

In 1972 the final Bachelor of Medicine and Surgery examinations were in two parts. The first part was clinical pathology which was taken six months before the final part. I have little memory of the pathology examination, but I clearly passed it without a problem and there was only one failure in our group.

The second part consisted of written papers and then clinical examinations and vivas. Except when seeing patients we dressed up in dinner jackets, bow tie and gown. This was known as *sub fusc* and was I think unique to Oxford. It is amazing that nearly 50 years on I can still remember to a very large extent the clinical examinations and in particular the vivas. The written papers in 1972 were indeed written – with short answers to the questions. Multiple choice questionnaires (MCQs), now very common and much easier to mark, had not come into the Oxford examination at that time. After my return from Zululand I had learned to use italic writing based on the marvellous script of Mr Anthony Barker (Chapter 7). I used the script in the examination, and this had an interesting effect in that because the writing was slower one had to think more clearly about what one wished to write down. The other surprising effect that it had was that I was commended by the examiners for my writing!

The clinical examination was in two parts and in four subjects. The main three subjects were medicine, surgery, and obstetrics and gynaecology. Each person taking the examination was then allocated to either anaesthetics, ear nose and throat, or ophthalmology on a random basis for a final short viva examination. In the three main subjects each student was given a long case and then a series of short cases. The long case examination consisted of taking a history from a patient, examining them, and then presenting the findings to the examiners, one external and one internal, followed by one's suggestions for diagnosis and treatment. The short cases consisted of anything between three and eight patients each with a simple and a solitary condition which we were then asked to diagnose and comment upon.

The medical long case I remember well. He was a patient with a neurological condition, and these are often the most difficult to examine particularly during a formal exam. One memory of this patient was testing his ankle reflexes. The common method is by tapping the Achilles tendon with a tendon hammer to see what reaction comes from the foot. During my time at Oxford I had been taught an alternate method of putting one's hand on the bottom of the foot and tapping one's own hand. This I did in front of the external examiner, who clearly had not seen the method before, and was suitably impressed by it. It turned out after a long discussion about the possible neurological problem of this patient that no diagnosis had been formally made, and the most probable diagnosis was multiple sclerosis. At least I felt better when I was told that my thoughts were reasonable but had not been formally confirmed.

My surgical long case was a young lad who had been having trouble passing urine and was having to do it more and more frequently and in small doses, normally something that happens with increasing age. He was known not to be a diabetic which was the most likely cause of the problem, and after examining the patient, looking at his x-rays and results, the answer became clear that he actually had tuberculosis of his bladder. A very uncommon diagnosis, and a little unfair in a final examination, but at least I had made the right diagnosis. For the short cases I was examined by Mr Taylor, a consultant orthopaedic surgeon who was the internal examiner. I had met Mr Taylor whilst I was a student doing a locum for the Accident Service. We had had a patient who was involved in a serious accident which needed both fixation of the fractures of his legs and the suturing of multiple facial lacerations. Mr Taylor fixed the fractures and I was still putting in several hundred sutures for the facial lacerations. Mr Taylor watched me for about three quarters of an hour as I finished, and afterwards his registrar said that he had never known Mr Taylor wait patiently for anything before. In the examination the first six or seven general surgical patients that I saw I was able to give a diagnosis, and clearly Mr Taylor had no further questions to ask (He was after all an orthopaedic surgeon). At last we came to a patient who had Dupuytren's contracture of his hand. An easy diagnosis to make, and at last Mr Taylor had some suitable questions. I passed the exam with ease.

The obstetrics and gynaecology examination was somewhat of a test. My internal examiner was Mr Arthur Williams, on whose firm I had been a student, and as I said earlier during that time we had not got on very well. In the viva his first question was extremely esoteric,

"What is an acardiac monster?" A diagnosis of which I had never heard, but luckily had enough Latin to translate. Clearly it had to be a child born without a heart, and amazingly during the viva I worked out that the only way this could happen was for identical twins to be sharing one placenta. One of the twins would have a functioning heart, the other would not, and the one with the heart would do the circulation for both the twins until they were born. I was feeling very happy with this diagnosis and then came his second, also esoteric, question,

"What is the hormonal treatment for Turner's syndrome?" Turner's syndrome is a rare abnormal chromosomal variation affecting female foetuses, and the patients as they grow, as well as having some physical differences to a normal person, are also unable to produce the normal female characteristic appearance and functions. They were then unable to have children, but this has now changed. The subject I had come across before and I was able to make some sensible comments. At that point the external examiner, the very famous Prof Dame Josephine Barnes took over. She had obviously realised that there had been problems between Arthur Williams and myself, and her first question was, "How long is a normal pregnancy?" I think Mr Williams got the message, and after that we went on to discuss more normal problems.

And then came the final and fourth part of the exam. Randomly I had been put in the group to be examined on ear nose and throat surgery. This was certainly my least popular of the three options, but clearly I did well enough to pass.

The Oxford final medical exam is unusual in that it did not classify people into grades as was normal in most exams, and in contrast to Cambridge, did not give a special honours award. I think that perhaps after my performance I would have deserved one, had one been available, but I may have been biased. Certainly the patients chosen were not at all simple for the level of a final examination, and later talking to people who did finals at other universities one realised just how esoteric were some of the diagnoses of the patients with which we were presented – but that was Oxford!

The results were announced the evening of the final vivas, and I, and all of my Oxford colleagues had passed. The only people that failed and had to redo the exam were people who had done their clinical work at other hospitals, mostly in London but were able to have taken the Oxford exam as they had taken their second MB exam at Oxford.

I then collected my degrees in the Sheldonian Theatre.

The two overseas study periods during my clinical years I have included here as two separate chapters.

SEVEN

UNIVERSITY OF THE WITWATERSRAND

During my time as a student I spent two periods studying in medical schools abroad. The first was in South Africa.

It is common at many medical schools for students in their penultimate or final year to have the opportunity to do elective studies. These can be either a period of research, or working at other medical schools in the United Kingdom or abroad, or working in hospitals in any part of the world. The normal period for the so-called elective is two or three months. I had already been offered a place at the Charles Johnson Memorial Hospital at Nqutu in Zululand South Africa. Two months would be a minimum useful period and having spent many hours and many weekends working in the Accident Department in Oxford, they agreed that I did not need to do my formal study period there, and I could have an extra month overseas. Also, by chance, although that sounds the wrong thing to say, I was going out on the odd occasion with the daughter of the professor of obstetrics and gynaecology. I met him at his house whilst I was studying for my two months in his department in Oxford. I discussed the possibility of adding an extra month to my elective, and his immediate question was,

"How many babies have you delivered?" I told him that the answer was seven and he agreed that if I delivered another three babies during my elective, I could have the extra month away. I very luckily managed to reorganise my flights and also to organise four months as a student at the University of the

Witswatersrand, with three of the months at the mission hospital in Zululand and the fourth month at Baragwanath Hospital in Soweto, the largest hospital in the Southern Hemisphere.

I made an effort to learn some basic Zulu language. Perhaps enough to say hello, or even better, to take a history from a patient. I knew that I was not a born linguist, and that certainly proved to be the case. One must remember that this was before the days of the internet, and although recordings were available, they were very expensive. Pronunciation is relatively simple as the language was written down by an Englishman and therefore one pronounces it as it is written. However, the exception is the three clicks, which I eventually learned after I had been there for some weeks, and can still do. The grammar is totally different to any other language that I had met, and it is based on the noun and not the verb. It is made even more confusing as there are no adjectives. It is quoted that the average intelligent English person has a vocabulary of 23,000 words but, without adjectives, the average Zulu herd boy needs 35,000 words. And the final problem is that in Zulu the only numbers are 1 to 10. Which means that a person who is 38 years old will tell you that he is tens that are three and ones that are eight. Now try a date!

It turned out that there was a scholarship available to me to pay for my flights. I went for an interview for this scholarship in London. I learned later that the money was from BOSS, the Bureau Of State Security. This was part of the South African government, and the interview was presumably to discover that I did not wish to go to South Africa to cause upset to the apartheid rule then present. I also received further small scholarships from the British Universities Society of Arts and from the British Medical Students' Trust. But at least they were more scholarships. The flight down was less traumatic than my first African flight to Zambia, and starting from Luxembourg entailed only one stop in Nairobi to refuel. I arrived in Johannesburg and caught a series of buses to arrive at Nqutu. The ride itself was interesting, and my first experience of apartheid. The last stage of the bus ride from Dundee to Nqutu was in a bus which was almost empty. I went to talk to the driver who told me that I was actually breaking the law because I was in the black part of the bus talking to him and not the white part where I should have been. We continued to talk. I arrived at the hospital to be greeted by one of the more remarkable people that I have ever met – Dr Anthony Barker. Anthony was a small man with a beard, a bow tie and a loud voice (Photo 7.1). Except in the operating theatre I don't think I ever saw him without his bow tie. I was shown

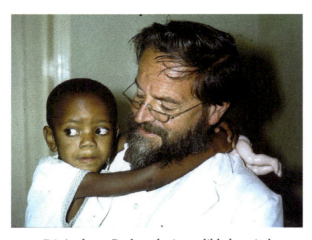

7.1 Anthony Barker, the incredible hospital superintendent, with a worried looking child and doll.

my quarters, a native rondavel which I was to share with another medical student, Jonty Ward from the Middlesex Hospital. Anthony then showed me around the hospital buildings, and I met his wife Dr Maggie Barker for the first time. Again a totally remarkable lady. The story of why they were in Zululand is told in Anthony's first book, *The Man Next to Me* which was re-issued as *Giving and Receiving*. In summary, Anthony had met Margaret when they were medical students at the University of Birmingham during the Second World War. She was studying medicine on a scholarship from the Church Missionary Society. During the war, Anthony had, as a conscientious objector, served as a doctor in the Merchant Navy on the Arctic convoys. At the end of the war Margaret was committed to working for three years for the missionary society at a hospital of their choice. She was allocated the Charles Johnson Memorial Hospital in Zululand. At this stage it had six beds. Rather than wait for two years for Maggie to return to England, and although Anthony was at that stage not a Christian, they decided to marry and to work together in the hospital in Zululand (Photo 7.2).

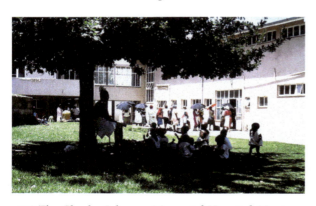

7.2 The Charles Johnson Memorial Hospital, Nqutu, KwaZulu. Sick and recovering children in front of the Children's Ward and the Maternity Department.

When I was there the hospital was situated in the small town of Nqutu. The town is situated in the North

West of Zululand, now KwaZulu Natal, some 40 miles from Vryheid and Dundee and 30 miles from a tarred road. The town consisted of a few shops, one hotel/bar, a prison and the hospital. The hospital was then a very major part of the town and had been increased enormously in size from when the Barkers had taken it on some 20 years earlier. Whenever the need arose for a new ward, Anthony would go somewhere around the World on a lecture tour and raise the money. From six beds it had grown to approximately 400 beds. The building and all of the maintenance was done locally. There had been established within it a nurse training school. The medical staff was Anthony and Maggie, four other doctors and six medical students (Photo 7.3). When I was there as a student four of these were from England and two from South Africa. There was also a physiotherapy student who was the daughter of one of the Barker relatives and whose father I had known as a doctor in Oxford. She later married one of the South African students. The head of the nursing school was Maggie's elder sister who had been a matron in England.

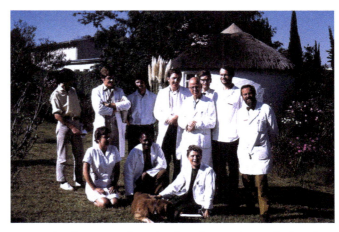

7.3 The doctors and medical students who worked and studied there in 1971 when I was a student.

As well as the wards, and two operating theatres, there was a mortuary and a large outpatient department. This latter was being run by an elderly retired GP from England, again a relative of the Barkers. Around Nqutu there were about eight outpatient stations which were set up on a fortnightly basis in small villages. One of these was at the famous battlefield of Isandlwana and another at Ulundi. where the Prince Imperial Napoleon had been killed in 1879.

I arrived on New Year's Eve 1970. With no chance to recover I was told that there was a dance that evening and we were all expected to perform with the nurses. As might be expected of Zulu ladies, they were all excellent dancers who mostly, because of the imbalance of numbers, were dancing with themselves. None of the male doctors or medical students had a single rest for a single dance all evening until the New Year was welcomed in.

The day that we had welcomed in was a Friday and I rapidly discovered my duties. There was a ward round at 8 o'clock every morning, and before this the two medical students on call either had to sew up the episiotomies and lacerations in the birth canal which were very common in the Zulu ladies caused by the babies born that night, or do any necessary post-mortems. Two of us were then allocated to go to the outpatient clinic within the hospital or to the clinic away from Nqutu in whichever village the doctor, nurses and ambulance were visiting that day. The remaining four students would be distributed between the two adult wards, the paediatric ward and the obstetric ward. When surgery was happening they would be assisting in theatre, often by giving the anaesthetic. One might have thought that the journey to some of the clinics would be a pleasant drive and with time to enjoy the magnificent scenery. This was definitely not the way that Anthony ran the hospital. As soon as we were in the back of the ambulance he would turn to the nurses and ask what would they like to be taught that day. The even worse news was that the medical student was the person who was to do the teaching with no prior warning as to the subject. And at the end of our teaching session Anthony would correct the errors and fill in the gaps that we had left. The clinics themselves were often very interesting and normally held in a store of some kind or a school. When we arrived there would be one hundred to two hundred patients awaiting in an orderly queue (Photo 7.4). To start with the students would listen, but very rapidly would be involved in seeing patients and doing such procedures as injections and removing teeth, there being no dentistry in the area. As a practical skill I found that learning to remove teeth, having given them a local anaesthetic beforehand was often a very interesting challenge. I do remember when I had been there some weeks asking Anthony why only two months later there were far more patients in the queue for tooth removal.

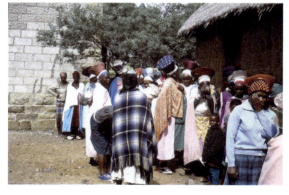

7.4 The queue at one of the peripheral clinics. This could be up to 300 patients.

He smiled and then told me how it was organised. All of the patients requiring a tooth removal would find the youngest person amongst them and put them near the front of the queue. If they came out having had a painless removal, the rest of the people waiting would remain in the queue, and if it had been a difficult or painful extraction then they would go away knowing that the following week there would be a different medical student. The number in the queue was therefore a simple measure of the ability of the student to give a good local anaesthetic and a painless removal. I must have removed some five hundred teeth, many of them rotten and in pieces, and that is far more than most dental students in the United Kingdom. One of the clinics was in the school on the site of the battle of Isandlwana. It is very impressive mountain. I tried to walk up the steep side on which the British army had been trapped, but it was remarkably unstable. I then discovered that I could walk up the back of the mountain, and I can claim to have climbed it. Talking to one of the Africans who was there acting as a guide I bought some of the bullets which had been fired by the British Army. They had been defeated because their replacement shells were locked away, and they could not open the cases in time. The Zulus had been told that no one dressed in red must survive, and that is exactly what happened. The only people who got away and walked or rode to Rorke's Drift were the engineers and other people who were not wearing red coats.

An interesting thing was that there were no records of the inpatients or of the outpatients within the hospital. Each patient had their own record card. If they had lost their record card, they were charged for another one, and virtually nobody came without their own card. A patient would pay ten cents for each visit. Anthony and Maggie had worked out that although the ten cents was a small amount, if people were made to pay something then they had a more complete belief in the treatment. I do wonder if the NHS in the United Kingdom should try the same method. If the patient was admitted the charge was one rand (about 5 shillings/25p) and this one rand would be the charge for one day, or for three months if that was necessary. The only people who were treated for nothing were those with TB, and their treatment was subsidised by the South African government. If the admission was for the birth of a baby, then the charge was five rand, but this would also include any treatment necessary for the child for their first year. This included vaccinations, and having paid for them, they were certainly going to have them. Because of this in the area of the Charles Johnson Hospital there was an incredibly low rate of measles, which can be a fatal disease among the Africans, and of diphtheria and of tetanus compared to the majority of the area of Zululand and probably South Africa. Tetanus in England is extremely rare but was common among the Zulus because the umbilical cord when it was cut was traditionally treated with cow dung. In the King Edward VII hospital in Durban there was a large ward full of babies with tetanus, many of whom succumbed to the disease.

Within the hospital Anthony did the surgery and much of the medicine. I once saw him do five surgical specialities on one list, two of them superbly and the other three very competently. For some reason the only thing that he was unhappy doing was ear, nose and throat surgery. Maggie was the paediatrician, and also a not very enthusiastic anaesthetist. She was competent but not an expert, and when I was there. there was no expert anaesthetist in the hospital. The obstetrics was divided between them, with Anthony doing the surgery and Maggie resuscitating and looking after the babies. Because of the lack of an anaesthetist and needing Maggie to look after the newborn, Anthony had devised a method of doing a caesarean section under local anaesthetic. I saw and learned to do the method and was extremely impressed with it. It has since spread around much of the developing world. One other advantage of the method is that the babies come out happily screaming as they have no general anaesthetic aboard. It is also a much safer method than doing an anaesthetic block of the spinal cord which as I saw later in Lesotho can spread up the spine to stop the lungs working and with a dead patient as the result.

Anthony was one of those amazing teachers of surgery. It is extremely difficult, as I was to discover later, to teach somebody an operation from the beginning of their practice. It is just so much easier to do it oneself with an assistant, but Anthony would take each of us through an operation doing a little bit at a time. By the end of a few weeks I was doing caesarean sections on my own, and also a variety of other operations. One that I remember was my introduction to plastic surgery. The Zulu women in the Bush often enlarge their earlobes for cosmetic reasons from a young age by making a small hole and then putting in increasing sizes of pieces of wood. These can often finish up some three inches in diameter. However when I was there it had become apparent that if they wanted a job in a town or city the fact they looked like country bumpkins – which they certainly were not – precluded them from work. Anthony therefore showed me how to correct this, and I became an expert at the operation of putting these enormous earlobes back to normal. Another patient I remember was somebody that had severely upset his wife and she had taken what in effect was a wooden hammer to his skull. He was brought into us bleeding from the scalp, but also with bone depressed into the brain and the fluid which normally surrounds the brain leaking out. I thought his time had come, and as Anthony was away at a clinic at the time. I took him to the operating theatre and cleared out the bone, repaired the layers of the linings of the brain and the skull, and closed the scalp. I thought that I had been wasting my time but about three days later a patient walking around the hospital came up to me and said thank you. To my amazement it was him. I had not recognised him at all, and it appeared that there was no permanent damage to his brain. Another patient had been stabbed in the chest and Anthony was again away from the hospital. None of the other doctors was willing to open the chest. We gave him the two units of blood that we had, but unfortunately his chest was still filling up. We therefore took the blood from around his lungs, mixed it with something to stop it clotting, and gave it back into a vein in his arm. At one point having taken some blood I gave it to Jonty Ward to crossmatch it. Jonty happily went off to the laboratories and came back about 10 minutes later and said,

"But it is his own blood." I'm afraid we all laughed. Jonty was a delightful character, but he did take nine years to complete a five-year medical course.

Teaching was not only on the wards, the operating theatres, and the outpatients but there was a weekly journal club where we took it in turns to present the results of papers published in the various journals. And we were 30 miles from a tarred road, and about 60 miles from the nearest hospital.

One field of medicine that was almost totally missing was psychiatry. When they first arrived the Barkers found that almost the only form of medical treatment was by the local witchdoctor. Slowly the patients started to come to the hospital as they realised that their treatment there was better. However the Barkers realised that the psychiatric treatment offered by the witchdoctor, the sangoma, was far better than anything that they could do. By the time that I was there, there was a simple arrangement that each swapped patients with the other as was relevant to the needs of that patient.

There was time off on Sundays, and often in the late afternoons. The hospital had a tennis court and a grass pitch on which softball was played. It is unbelievable now, but in the days of apartheid it was illegal for blacks and whites even to play sport together. In theory therefore we could not play with the nurses, but the hospital totally ignored the rules and we survived. I had some excellent games of tennis, which I normally lost, with one of the local lads who had been the black Zulu junior champion.

Anthony would have fun with the regulations. The Bantu Affairs Department (BAD) personnel were known as the BADDIES. When a junior BADDIE appeared to assess the hospital, Anthony would invite them in to watch an operation. However he would always pick a revolting, smelly, ghastly operation knowing that they had a fair chance of fainting. They would then be put in a bed on the male ward, which was of course for blacks, and when they awoke from their faint he would tell them that they were breaking the law, but of course there was no other way of treating them. They rarely gave a bad report of the hospital. And certainly without the restraints of apartheid I would have become involved with one of the nurses, a lovely lass called Futhie Ngema, which means 'it's a girl again'. Her father was the local vicar, and a fourth daughter was obviously too many for him.

We had two weekends away, one was to the game parks of Umfolozi and Hluhluwe, both magnificent and the oldest game parks in the whole of Africa. The second weekend was to Rorke's Drift where the famous battle of 1879 took place after the defeat of the British Army at Isandlwana which had been the only time that the British army was defeated by an army that had no guns. In Africa one has to be very careful about swimming in water as one can catch bilharzia. However, the water in the river Tugela is flowing rapidly enough that the bilharzia parasite cannot exist in it. Having seen the water, and desperately wanting a swim, I started to swim across Rorke's drift which looked very smooth. Halfway across I realised that I was being swept towards the waterfall and swam more rapidly, and survived. Leading up to the battle of Rorke's drift some of the people escaping from Isandlwana had been drowned swimming across the river but that was at the time of heavy rain and not the quiet period in which I was doing it. On another weekend two of the doctors invited me to go with them to Lourenco-Marques in Mozambique. Unfortunately I could not afford the fuel and the visa, and so it is still a country for me to visit.

As I said earlier the Barkers were two of the most remarkable people that I have ever met. Anthony was the front man and Maggie, when one got to know her, which was much more difficult, was clearly the strength behind the pair. They had taken on a challenge as young doctors, and over the years had established one of the great teaching hospitals, certainly in Africa, and perhaps throughout all developing countries. They had no children and the pressures upon them were therefore different to many couples. They had also passed their necessary examinations from the bush with neither of them having worked in the United Kingdom. Anthony had the Fellowship of the Royal College of

Surgeons and a Doctor of Medicine degree by thesis. He was later made a CBE, which I still think was rather unfair on Maggie. Maggie became a member of the Royal College of Obstetrics and Gynaecology. As a matter of principle they had never accepted a penny from the South African government, and they were living on, if I remember correctly, £320 a year from the Mission Society. There was virtually no pension due to them, and therefore when they were fifty five they decided to return to England to work for the National Health Service for ten years. They were offered various jobs and Anthony decided to become the first accident and emergency consultant at St George's Hospital in London. Within eighteen months he had passed the membership examination of the Royal College of Physicians by examination. A remarkable feat. They were loaned the money to buy a small flat in Wimbledon and furnished this themselves. At one time Anthony had noticed that they were removing some teak floorboards from the hospital and on enquiring what was to happen to the floorboards discovered that they were to be burned. He took them home and made the furniture for their flat. As well as working in the hospital they were both very involved in the racial problems around Tooting where the hospital was situated. They retired at age 65 as was then the requirement of the NHS. A few years later they were celebrating their golden wedding by riding their tandem around the Lake District as a repeat of their honeymoon. They were hit by a lorry and both killed. It may have been the best thing for them, as if they had died separately, the one remaining would have been totally lost.

I had arranged to have the last week of the three months free before moving to Johannesburg. During this week I first hitched to Durban and spent three days there with a doctor that I had known in Oxford. My main memory of the hospital was a very large room with an oblong bench in the middle. During the wet season of the year diarrhoea and vomiting was a very major and serious problem in young babies. A baby would be brought in severely dehydrated, and if possible a cannula was put into one of the veins of the scalp and fluid given. There were up to two hundred babies in this ward and they would be there between 24 and 48 hours. The scalp veins were inserted by specially trained and very expert technicians. If they failed there was clearly no point in us trying, and we would then do what was called a venous cut down and put the cannula into a major vein close to an ankle. And that was quite a challenge in a small dehydrated baby. After my three days in Durban I hitchhiked to Cape Town. People giving lifts were extremely generous, and often offered me a bed in their house. I remained in touch with one family for several years afterwards

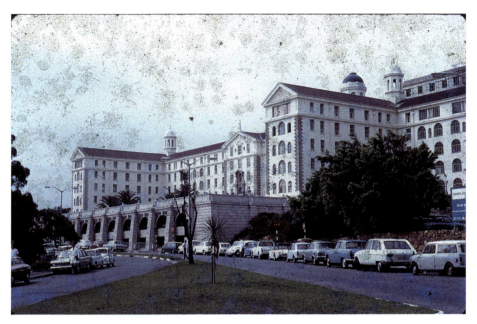

7.5 Groote Schuur Hospital in Cape Town where I watched the famous heart transplant surgeon Christiaan Barnard performing an operation.

and they also stayed with us in England. I can remember one other lift when I was picked up by a gentleman who was Dutch. He and his family had gone to live in South Africa after the second world war. Talking to him I discovered that he had two daughters, one of whom was a medical doctor and the other had a PhD. I asked him what language they spoke at home. His answer was that their first choice was Dutch, their second choice English, and when they had to, they spoke Afrikaans, or as he called it kitchen Dutch.

In Cape Town I had a contact with Sarah Yates, a nurse who had been one of the cooks in the Murison Small ski chalet in which I had stayed in Verbier. She put me up for some three days. She was working as a theatre sister in cardio-thoracic surgery, and organised for me to watch the famous Christiaan Barnard, the heart transplant surgeon, whom I had met in Cambridge, operate in Groote Schuur Hospital (Photo 7.5). I then took two days to hitchhike the eight hundred miles to Johannesburg via the famous Kimberley Diamond fields and the Rhodes Museum. On this journey a Rhodesian student and myself at one time were given a lift together by an Afrikaans diplomat who was on leave at home. As we passed through Potchefstroom, an absolute hotbed of Afrikanaarism, he said that much as he would like a cup of coffee, if he stopped

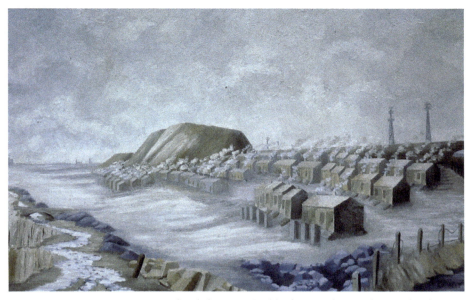

7.6 Soweto. During apartheid this was the black township to the south of Johannesburg. Attached was Baragwanath Hospital, the largest in Africa and the third largest in the world. I studied there in 1971. The painting is by Gill Scott (now Pittman). She also studied there and 50 years later we remain friends.

with the two of us in the car he would be lynched. We were not sure if he was joking.

For my last month I was officially a member of the University of the Witwatersrand and was based at the famous Baragwanath Hospital in Soweto just to the south of Johannesburg. Soweto (SOuth WEst TOwnship) was the black township for the area during the days of apartheid (Photo 7.6). The hospital had 3500 beds, and often considerably more patients. It was very famous for the trauma work that it did, which was very necessary both in Soweto and the neighbouring districts. I joined one of the surgical teams which was under the leadership of Prof H H Lawson. There was one registrar and two housemen (recently qualified doctors) as well as two students from Johannesburg and myself making up the firm. Prof Buddy Lawson's team was one of three teams and we were therefore on-call every third day and night. It was incredibly busy, especially on every Friday night which was the local pay day, when the rate both of drunkenness and trauma went up very considerably. The last Friday of the month was even worse, and when I was there we had 80 acute surgical admissions for trauma as well as the more routine surgical emergencies.

This was the time of rigid apartheid which had been largely ignored at Nqutu. I immediately fell foul of this when I met one of the nurses who had been at Nqutu, and we gave each other a gentle hug. I was told that it was definitely not acceptable. And a few days later during a lunch break, I asked where one of the junior doctors on our team had gone. A slightly awkward silence and I was then asked if I had not realised that he was coloured, and therefore had to eat in a separate mess.

Of the students I was the most experienced, particularly from my previous three months in Nqutu and my earlier experience both in Zambia and in Oxford. I started as all students do by being assessed when I was seeing patients and assisting at operations. Very soon I was doing the operations on my own, and at one stage Prof Lawson was asked to go to see the medical director who suggested to him that a medical student working on his own was not acceptable. Prof Lawson very rapidly put him right. I therefore continued doing surgery on my own.

It is normal practice for anyone that has been stabbed in the abdomen to be taken to theatre to have the wound explored to make sure that no deep damage had been done. With the enormous amount of trauma coming through the unit, with up to 10 or 15 abdominal wounds on a busy night, this was simply not possible. A new test had been devised where a litre of normal saline was run into the abdomen through a needle, and the bottle then put on the floor to see what came back. If it was clear the needle was removed, the wound on the skin was sutured and the patient put to bed for the night for continuing assessment. If they were well the next morning, and remembering the enormous pressure on beds, the patient was asked to stand up, and if this was satisfactory to walk towards the door. If they got to the door without looking in difficulty or in pain he continued to walk and was effectively discharged. The original idea of the litre in and litre out was known then as the Baragwanath test, and is now called a Diagnostic Peritoneal Lavage (DPL), although in developed countries now rarely used as it has been superseded by ultrasound scans. We named the 'walking test the next morning' the second Baragwanath test. I do not think that it has spread around the world. If the litre that came out of the patient's abdomen was either at all bloody or with any obvious faecal material within it, then the patient was taken to the operating theatre for a standard laparotomy where the abdomen was opened, the damage assessed and repaired.

The other common problem was stab wounds to the chest and to the heart. Baragwanath Hospital had an incredible reputation for dealing with these stab wounds. If the patient came in alive, it was a standard registrar's operation to open the chest and repair the damage. 96% of the patients who came in alive, left alive. If the stab wound had damaged the lungs causing a pneumothorax, where air is inappropriately situated between the lungs and the rib cage, then a chest drain was inserted. In South Africa this was a routine student's procedure, and my record was 23 chest drains put in on one night. In the whole of my career I doubt if I have put in a further 23, and very few medical students in England would have put in one.

In those days, with a white coat and a stethoscope around my neck, I could walk around Soweto at night and be totally protected. I understand now that a doctor cannot walk from one end of the hospital to the other without an armed guard. Fights were between the tribes and very rarely involved people of another race. Before I was there, there had been a terrible way of stealing money, particularly on the trains which were packed with people tightly packed and standing. A sharp screwdriver or stiff wire would be used to push in through the skin of the back and paralyse the person by transecting their spinal cord. This of course left them permanently paralysed, and when I arrived there were three wards full of these people in their wheelchairs. The government solved the problem by making a mandatory death sentence for anyone using the method.

Back to Oxford I went as a much more experienced student and with a deep love of Africa and Africans, especially the Zulus. Very soon after I returned I met Prof Stallworthy.

"Did you deliver your three babies?" was his first question. I said that I had done three Caesers on my own, and at the look on his face, I thought that I had better tell him about the other sixty odd ordinary deliveries that I had also done.

EIGHT

UNIVERSITY OF MICHIGAN

At the University of Oxford medical school all students had the option of spending two months doing an elective. This had to involve medical work or study and different people did a variety of electives, from doing research to spending a period in a specific department either in Oxford or anywhere in the UK, or studying or doing a placement in a hospital abroad. The elective did not need to be in a university environment and my elective had been in South Africa. In addition to this two months, as long as one was going to a recognised university department of medicine we could study away from Oxford for any part, or parts of the degree course. What a brilliantly enlightened attitude which I think was then unique in any British medical school. One friend in my year, Shelagh Doherty, spent nine months in various overseas attachments.

There was advertised a travelling scholarship to Iowa University in the States for which I competed, but was beaten into second place by a fellow student Peter Teddy. I was therefore looking around for another option. By chance long term friends of mine had moved to Ann Arbor in Michigan and they very kindly offered me their spare bedroom. Paediatric teaching in Oxford did not then have a good reputation and I contacted the department at the famous University of Michigan. By return of post I was offered a place for two months. I would have to become a registered student, but the fee was remarkably small. I therefore contacted my friends Tony and Meg Atkins and arranged to go to them for October and November 1971.

I had two other contacts in the States at the time and I planned to spend two weeks seeing other parts of the country on my way to Michigan. Peter Burgess had been a flatmate in London when I was lecturing at the University of Surrey and he and his wife had emigrated to New Jersey four years previously. The other contact was a British neurosurgeon who was spending some years in Kentucky and was a friend of a girlfriend, Christine Harrington, in London.

I flew to New York by Pan-Am and had an interesting experience in the plane. I had just started going out with my future wife, Vivian, and was writing to her with my (then) immaculate italic writing. This was noticed by an air hostess who was clearly astounded, and who then borrowed my letter to show to all her colleagues. Luckily there was nothing embarrassing within it. Clearly italic writing did not exist in the States. On arrival in the morning, I had the usual American problems with immigration and customs. I had my bags searched for the only time in all of my international travels – then or since, but life became easier when they found my stethoscope and discovered that I was a medical student arriving to study. I was met by Peter and we spent the day in the city visiting the Empire State Building and taking a boat to see the Statue of Liberty. We then drove to his house in Trenton, just across the border in New Jersey where I spent two days with Peter and his wife, whose best man I had been at their wedding. I then took the train to Philadelphia which I found more impressive than New York with the old buildings, the Liberty Bell, Independence Hall and a museum which were all well worth seeing. Walking around the city I also felt more relaxed than I had been in New York.

Being a poor medical student, the next parts of my journey were by Greyhound Bus with the ticket costing 99 dollars. The journey to Louisville in Kentucky took about 15 hours, and with careful timing the journey was also used for sleeping during the night. On arrival I was met by the neurosurgeon who was a complete stranger to me. We immediately established a friendship and I stayed in their house for the next three days. The first two days were a fascinating introduction to medicine in the States, and to medical education there. John had been living and working there for, I think, about three years, and was certainly unimpressed by the medical training. All medical students had already studied for a first degree, in a science, and must have done well to be accepted onto a medical degree course. The course there was incredibly competitive as the marks obtained were almost the only guide to career progression. John was telling me that in a laboratory one student would intentionally upset a piece of apparatus to make it more difficult for the next student to use. A total difference to England where, I think without exception, we all helped each other, and particularly the weaker members of our year. I also remember that he told me that when he was examining in an anatomy exam, that the level of knowledge was far below that of an equivalent student in England. Tragically, as in so many other things, we have now followed the States, and examining and teaching that I now do, I find that the level of anatomy is far below the standard when I qualified. The excuse now is that they have spent more time learning how to talk to a patient. Somehow that seemed to be built in automatically in my time.

On the third day there his senior trainee, and very obviously a rich young man and a Kentucky Colonel, took us all to the Country Club for lunch. Again an introduction to a very different life that a normal tourist would never see. The honorary rank of Colonel is very American, and is bestowed on people by State Governors officially on people doing good works, but I think donations to election expenses may be more important. In Kentucky in the 1970s, the Governor was creating 10,000 Colonels a year. That afternoon we all drove to the state border with Ohio and were standing on a railway bridge when a train came past. The incredible shaking of the bridge was something still in my memory!

With a twelve hour Greyhound trip to Ann Arbor via Detroit I was both able to save the cost of another night's accommodation, and also to visit the Ford factory in Detroit. Having spent six weeks working in the Ford factory in Dagenham this was indeed a very interesting contrast. And finally to Ann Arbor where I was met by Meg and Tony Atkins with whom I took up residence in their rented two bedroom one story house about three miles north of the centre of the town and the hospital. Very luckily it was well heated as the temperature was well below zero. I had known Meg for some six years and we had been close friends for one of them. After Meg and I had parted as boy and girlfriend we had remained very good friends, and she had met Tony on one of the ski holidays that I had organised. They had subsequently married. Tony I had met when we were both engineering research students at Cambridge. He had started his career in industry and the year before I stayed with them moved into academia, and in fact stayed there for his working life and finished as the last Professor of Engineering at Reading University. Very sadly after he retired that University dropped engineering from the available courses. During my stay with them I discovered new things about Tony. He had been a percussionist in the Welsh National Youth Orchestra, and was still involved in music. He was also very involved in bringing Isambard Brunel's ship 'SS Great Britain' back from the Falklands, where it was rotting, to Bristol and where it now proudly floats. He had also written, and continued to write, books about the Great Western Railway on which he was an acknowledged expert. He died in 2018. Meg remains a close friend.

I settled in over the weekend and on the Monday morning, in the dark and freezing cold, I borrowed Tony's bike and rode downhill to the Hospital. Having somewhat unfrozen I discovered the department of paediatrics (pediatrics in American English) and found Dr Richard Allen. He was the attending (consultant) doctor in pediatric neurology, and had two training doctors working with him. He was about 15 years older than me, quite small and with a pronounced limp from a cause that I did not discover, and he was very welcoming. (As an aside I have noticed that very often male paediatricians around the world are often quite short.) We discussed what he expected of me – which actually was very little, for the reason that I was to discover very shortly – and I suggested to him what I would like to gain from the visit.

To make more sense of the next part a background to the town, to the university and to the medical school would be helpful. Ann Arbor was established in 1824 and was named after the wives, both Ann, of the founding fathers. The wives had become involved with a local patch or arbor of oak trees. The town grew slowly until 1837 when the University of Michigan moved there from Detroit, and it then grew very rapidly. When I was there in the 1970s the population was approximately 100,000 of which nearly 30,000 were employed by the university or hospital. In addition there were about 30,000 students in the university. In England at that time only the University of London with its multiple colleges was approaching that number, and most universities had between 2,000 and 6,000 students. The University of Michigan is a public university, and not to be confused with the Michigan State University situated in East Lansing. It ranks in the top 25 universities in the USA. The medical school has 2,000 students and is ranked fifth in the United States. The hospital in 1971, when I was there, was in one large building, but in 2011 the department of pediatrics moved into the new CS Mott's Children's Hospital with 240 beds.

In the 1970s medicine in the States was very different to that in the United Kingdom. In Britain then, a patient was under the care of one consultant, and if necessary they would be transferred for special expertise to the care of another colleague, within the hospital or in another hospital. In the States a patient could be under the simultaneous care of several consultants and definitive decisions were made more difficult, and often delayed. Unfortunately the

UK is beginning to follow this method. But the major difference was money. In clinics in Michigan I regularly heard the attending doctor say to a parent that if they would allow their child to be entered into a research programme then the treatment was free, and as medicine was all private there was a major inducement, if not an absolute requirement, for this to happen. In those days I had not been involved with Ethical Committees and did not find out what the situation there was. But there was certainly no shortage of patients for research studies.

What surprised me most about the medical students was that they were almost never seen on the wards, which explained why Dr Allen thought that he would have little input into my stay. Not living in student accommodation, I met almost no medical students. It became apparent that they were not on the wards because the medical degree examinations were about basic knowledge and had almost no clinical component or patient examination requirements. Having come from the system in England, my interest was not in multiple lectures, but in doing ward rounds and attending out-patient clinics. I was therefore extremely welcome and very soon was doing the routine clinics almost on my own, with the doctors there to offer advice when needed. Dr Allen's research, which was internationally recognised, was studying the effects of metabolic diseases on the nervous system. This was a small part of the work of the unit in which epilepsy affected the majority of the patients. Many of these were resistant to treatment and were extremely serious, having a terrible effect on the children, their families, and on all of us in the hospital. I remember two cases (a terrible word but it usefully includes the children and the families) from the clinics. The first was a child who after examination clearly had a common cold. Having told the parents this, I asked why they had brought the child to the paediatric clinic in the hospital.

"An out-patient clinic visit is much cheaper than going to our family doctor." A suitable explanation, and they probably also had a better examination and service.

The second patient was a young child with classical but moderate epilepsy who had attended many times before. After the examination I told the parents that the diagnosis was epilepsy and gave them details of the disease and the treatment and I was amazed when they replied,

"Thank you very much. That is what we thought, but no doctor has ever told us the diagnosis."

Out of interest I did attend some M and M conferences at 8am on Saturdays.

These Morbidity and Mortality conferences were in theory a chance to find out what had caused medical problems and their possible solution in the future. Unfortunately they turned out to be a chance for junior doctors to show off their knowledge, or perhaps their recent reading, and score points against their rivals. It was typical for one of them to quote a particularly obscure paper in a journal of which no one had heard, and then blame their colleague for not having read it. The one case that I do remember was a report by a visiting British junior surgeon about the terrible things that had happened to a patient having been pricked by a needle. Much to the amusement of the few British people present it turned out that the patient was the presenting doctor who had scratched himself and he had written his very amusing presentation about a non-existent problem. The locals were not at all amused, humour was clearly not allowed.

Another difference between the two medical schools was the almost complete lack of any social communication between doctors and students. I never talked to the doctors about anything except work, even when I spent a considerable time with them doing EEGs (electro-encephalograms) on the children. The only social contact that I had was with the dietician in the unit. We had presumably talked about my previous career, and she mentioned that her husband was a director of the pharmaceutical giant Smith and Nephew. They very kindly invited me to join their family for Thanksgiving, the great American event, on the 25th of November.

Life was not as boring as the impression I may have given because staying with Tony and Meg who had made local friends, and from his British tradition he also had his students regularly to the house. Talking to a student after a concert in which Tony was performing, I asked her about her interest in music, and was astonished to discover that her interest arose because she received extra marks towards her engineering degree for her involvement. Tony and Meg were extremely generous and at weekends we would tour the local country, although it was covered in deep snow. We went to an American Football game which went on for far too long, especially as the temperature was below freezing, and was very boring for someone who was not a supporter of one of the teams. We also went to a performance of Handel's Messiah where the hundreds of the audience were all handed a detailed copy of the music on entry and encouraged to join in, especially in the Hallelujah Chorus – a memorable event indeed. I also discovered the university ice hockey club, with whom I did some training and then played for the medics' team against the engineers. We won easily, but what did surprise me was the relatively low standard of the players, many of whom had been brought up in the cold state of Michigan. Having always been second or third choice in England, to suddenly being clearly the best player on the ice was a very pleasant surprise.

After two months of American medicine the summary of my feelings was that I did not like it, and it made me far far more appreciative of the NHS, even with its failings and problems. When later in my career I had the choice of spending a year back in the States or going to Australia, my decision was very simple. Australia.

NINE

HOUSE OFFICER

BATTLE HOSPITAL, READING LOCUM SENIOR HOUSE OFFICER

I collected my degrees of Bachelor of Medicine and Bachelor of Surgery in the Sheldonian Theatre in Oxford and then Vivian and I had a short proper honeymoon in France touring the Chateaux of the Loire and camping *au sauvage*, returning home at the end of June.

In the good old days when one had passed one's final examination and graduated one could immediately start working as an independent doctor. When I qualified in 1972, to become a fully registered independent doctor one had to do one year of hospital appointments. At the end of the year, if the two consultants with whom one was registered agreed to sign one up, and say that one was as brilliant as was expected of a fully registered doctor, one could then practice with no one looking over one's shoulder to make sure that one was safe. The position now, in 2021, is that the qualified doctor has to spend two years in several recognised posts before becoming fully registered.

From my Cambridge preclinical days, I had been offered my surgical six-month house job with Mr John Withycombe at Addenbrookes hospital in Cambridge (Photo 9.1). With that job organised the problem then was that the job did not start until October, and I therefore had three months free. Rather than take an extended holiday I decided to look for a locum post to earn some money and to get more experience. Throughout the next few years, I always felt that I should do as many locum posts as possible as my age made me feel that

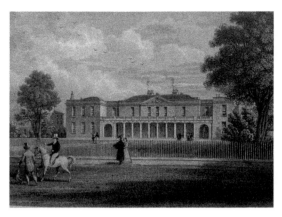

9.1 Addenbrooke's Hospital, Cambridge 1870

I should try to catch up with those who were ten years younger than me, but had qualified at the same time.

I do not know how I heard of it but there was a locum in orthopaedics and casualty needed at the Battle Hospital in Reading. I went for an interview with Mr Chesterman who immediately said that I could start the next week. I pointed out to him that as I was not registered I was not allowed to work on my own in casualty. He basically said that with my Oxford degree I would be far better than any other locum that might come his way, and I should simply ignore the official regulation. Mr Chesterman was an interesting character who some months later appeared in the national newspapers. A postman had come to see him in the outpatient clinic. Mr Chesterman having discovered that the man was on strike at the time said that so was he, and the patient could come back to the outpatients after he had returned to work. I think this went up to the General Medical Council, and somehow Mr Chesterman did keep his licence.

Vivian was still working in Oxford, and we were living there except when I had to stay in a room at the Battle Hospital on my on-call nights when she would sometimes join me in the single bed when she was not herself on call. On the return from our second honeymoon I therefore arrived at the Battle Hospital on the monday morning to be shown round, to meet the other two consultant orthopaedic surgeons, Mr Squire and Mr Scott, the operating theatre and ward sisters, and the staff of the accident and emergency department. Mr Squire was a marvellous old-time orthopaedic consultant who was absolutely delightful. He had played rugby for Richmond and at county level for Devon in his younger days. Mr Scott was very different. He was also very pleasant but not the extrovert character of the other two. He had worked in the Sudan for some years and as I was to discover over the next few months he was somewhat out of date.

And so to work – and back to earning money after four years.

Reading had two main hospitals. The Royal Berkshire was a magnificent Regency building and thought itself to be far more important than the Battle

Hospital situated at the other end of the town. The Battle Hospital had originally been opened as a workhouse in 1867. During the first world war it became the Reading War Hospital and then in 1938 changed its name again to the Battle Hospital. In 1972 a large single story hospital was added, and this was to be the trial of the design of future hospitals in Britain. Clearly it was not a success as it closed in 2005, and all of the patients were moved to the Royal Berkshire Hospital. The orthopaedic wards, the orthopaedic operating theatres and the accident and emergency department were all in the old part of the hospital.

Although I had been extremely fortunate in being allowed to do a large amount of surgery in Oxford, even more was now thrown my way. Before I arrived the nurses in the casualty department did most of the suturing. I think they were happy that I changed this, and I did the suturing, particularly of any facial wounds. I was also correcting many of the fractures and started to learn the technique of pinning fractures of the neck of the femur. The staffing levels were very different to those of a major teaching hospital. There was a marvellous consultant anaesthetist who worked with the orthopaedic team, and he would jokingly tell us that he was about to do a ward round of his patients – normally done on a ward when all the patients are visited in turn. The usual way to give an anaesthetic is that the anaesthetist, often with an assistant, would be looking after one patient at a time. Not the Reading anaesthetist, who would have one patient going to sleep in the anaesthetic room, one patient asleep in each of the two operating theatres, and the fourth one waking up in the recovery room. And in the months that I was there, there was never a problem.

With my experience of neurosurgery at Oxford, I had probably done more operating on skulls than any of the three consultants. On one occasion I was assisting Mr Scott with an operation for a severely fractured skull. After about two minutes of removing odd pieces of bone he asked me what he should do next. From my experience, but with some trepidation I gave him my advice, at which point he handed over the operation to me to complete, which I managed to do successfully. Another patient that I remember was a young teenager who had been hit on the head and knocked unconscious. When he was brought into casualty I examined him and it was clear that he needed to be transferred to the neurosurgery unit in Oxford as he had a potentially serious bleed within his skull. I phoned the registrar on call who immediately said to send him over urgently. Mr Chesterman was just behind me at the time, and after the young lad had departed said to me that it normally took him half an hour of argument before they would accept the transfer of a patient and wondered how

I had done it. Implying, but not actually saying it, that they knew that I could carry out an accurate neurological examination, I said,

"I have worked there, Sir."

There was a social life which was well organised by Mr Squire. We dined with him and his wife, and he was also president of the local lawn bowls club. There was a challenge between his team from the hospital, where most of us had never tried bowls before, against his club. The amazing result was that we won, and I still cannot imagine how or why.

It was an enjoyable and worthwhile three months. I learned a lot, had a lot of experience, and hopefully contributed usefully to the Department. I am pleased to say that there was no comeback to the fact that I was actually working there illegally on many occasions when I would send the patient home without being seen by a fully registered doctor.

ADDENBROOKE'S HOSPITAL, CAMBRIDGE HOUSE SURGEON

In October the Cambridge job was due to start. My wife, Vivian, also needed a six-month appointment as part of her general practice qualification. A post in dermatology in which she was interested went to a local Cambridge man, and she took a post in radiotherapy which was based in the new Addenbrooke's Hospital about 1½ miles away from the city centre. My post started with Mr John Withycombe who was a full-time urological surgeon in the old Addenbrooke's Hospital (Photo 9.2). I had been very pleased to discover that the six-month job was to be three months of urology and then three months of general surgery with Mr Everett. This would give me a far better introduction to surgery. Two of us had been appointed to the job which we shared between us. The other doctor was a fully registered doctor, Dr Tim Walsh, an outstanding man who had already won the Hallett prize for the best performance throughout the country in the first part of the fellowship examination of the Royal College of Surgeons of England. It turned out that we would not only share the same job, but we were both offered married flats on the same landing of No 1, Trumpington Street, a very attractive Georgian building attached to the hospital and with a view overlooking Hobson's Conduit.

The problem with urology was that although very common, most of the surgery for prostatic disease was done by the surgeon through a cystoscope and there was no need for an assistant. The only operations where an assistant was essential were removing a kidney or operating on the bladder, particularly for cancer. The workload for the junior houseman was on the ward and was extremely busy clerking the large number of elderly patients who needed surgery, and often had multiple medical or surgical problems. I always went to the operating theatre if for no other reason than to hear Mr Withycombe's stories and jokes. He was the most delightful person, and normally got on well with everybody. There was however one theatre sister who had clearly upset him. In the tearoom he had told us the rhyme about the nurses of the London hospitals. The part of this that I remember was 'Guys for wives, Barts for tarts and at St Thomas's for young ladies.' When we went back into the theatre Mr Withycombe asked the theatre sister,

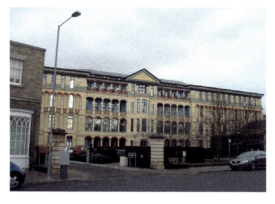

9.2 Addenbrooke's Hospital. The buildings which were in the courtyard when I was a student and was working there have now been removed. It is now the Judge Business School.

"Sister, where did you train?"

"St Bartholomew's Hospital." was the answer at which he turned to us and said,

"Can't you tell." Sister never did discover why we all fell about laughing. On another occasion a policeman had remonstrated with him as he had cycled on the footpath from his home to the hospital. Mr Withycombe told him that it was much safer cycling on the footpath and as the speed at which he cycled was the same as the pedestrians, surely he could be doing no harm. The outcome of the debate we did not discover.

At the beginning of the term Dr Wright, the anatomy Fellow from Clare College, had asked me whether I would like to supervise anatomy for undergraduates from Newham College and Trinity Hall. I said that I would be delighted to do so. I then asked Mr Withycombe whether, one or two at a time, my students would be allowed into the operating theatre to see some real surgery. He said he would be delighted for that to happen, but I had to understand that if they couldn't answer his anatomical questions, then he would ask me to do so. Slightly worrying, but it worked out very well. He was an examiner both for the University of Cambridge and for the Royal College of Surgeons but had the slightly unfortunate soubriquet of 'smiling death'.

One of the most useful techniques that I learned was catheterising elderly gentleman who had been unable to pass water because of their prostatic disease. This can often be very difficult and appeared to happen much more often in the middle of the night than in daytime. If the light on the ward went on in the small hours of night, very often would appear a particular senior nurse. She was the most marvellous lady who had been the urology ward sister for many years. It had then been made clear to her that unless she took promotion, nurses that she had trained would be in charge of her. She took the promotion, but being a single lady remained living in the nurses' home, and the light coming on in 'her' ward would instantly bring her to the ward, where she was extremely welcome and very helpful.

An unusual additional part of this job was to be on the cardiac resuscitation team with the role of anaesthetic assistant. On the occasions when the duty anaesthetist had been called to the maternity hospital some miles away, we were expected to take over the anaesthetic role. Having qualified in Oxford and worked in Africa this was only slightly worrying to me, but very frightening for the house surgeons coming from the London hospitals, rarely with any previous experience. For the first three or four weeks they spent as much time as they could learning, and getting experience in anaesthetics. The worst part about it for me was that it was on the second floor of the main hospital. I remember one night where there were three arrests on the cardiac unit. My first floor flat was about 200 yards away from the bottom of the steps, and I then had to run-up three floors three times as the lift was not on the ground floor when I arrived. I was suitably exhausted at the end, but at least the patient survived.

After three months Tim Walsh and I swapped jobs. The second post was house surgeon to Mr Bill Everett, who was a delightfully quiet man and a brilliant surgeon. I learned there that to judge the excellence of a surgeon one only had to look to see if his colleagues came to them for their own operations. And it was certainly the case for Mr Everett. The team consisted of David Dunn as the senior registrar, David Drake as the registrar and myself as the house surgeon. Both the Davids were relatively senior in their roles, and Mr Everett exposed me to as much surgery as was possible. At night we shared the duties with Prof Roy Calne's team. In theory it was a one in two on-call rota, but the weekly teaching session by Prof Calne was at 9 o'clock on the Saturday morning. I well remember one day when a junior surgeon about to take the fellowship exam was asked to examine and present a patient to Prof. Prof then said,

"After what you have just told me, should I take any notice of what you have said?" A very chastened junior. Prof then demonstrated to us all how it should be done. A lesson that I have not forgotten.

For those of us who wished to be surgeons attendance at this was essential, and as Mr Everett's operating list was on a Monday morning, I also had to clerk all of the patients on the Sunday afternoon whether I was on-call or not. The longest time I therefore had free in my three months was about 26 hours. I was clearly learning to be a surgeon because my time off in the future was rarely more than that until my retirement. How life has changed for modern junior trainee surgeons with EU 48hr regulations There was one downside to the post for somebody wishing to be a surgeon, and that was that Mr Everett had only one complication during my three months that I worked for him. Marvellous for the patients, but less good for a junior trainee surgeon who needed to learn about complications and their treatment. Very soon I was doing the appendicectomies on my own after discussing the case with one of the Davids. I do remember one young PhD student with a severe appendicitis who I examined, and then telephoned David Drake who told me to get on with it. I operated and removed a classical inflamed appendix. The next day on the ward round Mr Everett greeted the patient by his Christian name and asked him what he was doing in the bed. He explained that his appendix had been taken out the previous night at which point Mr Everett turned to me and said,

"Was it a classic appendicitis?" To which I could honestly say yes.

"Well done," he said. What the young lad had not told me was that he was actually the son of Mr Everett's next-door neighbours. On another occasion Mr Everett looked at the operating lists to see what he was going to be operating on, and then told David Dunn to assist David Drake, whilst he would assist me. A marvellous way of learning the technique of operating. One other patient that I remember was a cancer of the oesophagus. This was to be removed by an ear, nose and throat surgeon, and at the same operation Mr Everett, with me assisting, was mobilising the stomach to bring it up to join with the upper part of the oesophagus which was clear of the cancer. At the top end of the operating table there was a lot of noise coming from the operating surgeon and a considerable amount of blood flowing everywhere. At our end of the table there existed a calmness, and the use of about five swabs to mop up the very minimal amount of blood that Mr Everett was spilling. A contrast between techniques from which I hopefully learned and used throughout my career.

I remember another patient who was well into his nineties and who had a large aortic aneurysm which had given him some pain from a small leak. Prof Calne came to see him and told him that without surgery he would die, and with an operation he had a 90% chance of dying. Prof then asked him,

"Do you want an operation?"

"Of course," came the reply. So he had his operation and did survive.

I had two near disasters during the three months. The first, and what could potentially have been a major disaster for me was an elderly gentleman who had been sent in with renal colic. I clerked him in the emergency admission room, gave him suitable analgesia for his pain and admitted him to the ward. I heard the next morning that he died during the night. The post-mortem showed that he had had a leaking aneurysm and not a stone in the ureter. Mr Everett consoled me by saying that the post mortem had shown that an operation would not have been possible in any case.

The second case was a young lad sent in with abdominal pain. On examination it was not classical of any obvious cause, and after some analgesia for his relief I sent him home. Twenty four hours later he was back with a classical appendicitis. I took it out and found that luckily it had not ruptured, and he recovered well.

I have said earlier that Cambridge undergraduates had to go to a different hospital to complete their clinical training. In 1972 the University began to trial clinical training for a very few people in Cambridge. One of these was a professor of chemistry who had retired at the age of 60 when he had decided to read medicine. In my engineering time in Cambridge I had been to some of his lectures, and it was interesting that I was now teaching him on the wards. His chemistry lectures had been interesting not only for the chemistry, but also for the presence of the Australian sub four minute miler and world record holder, Herb Elliott. What he was doing in Cambridge at the time I never did discover.

BATTLE HOSPITAL, READING HOUSE PHYSICIAN

I had been incredibly lucky to have been offered the Cambridge post, but it was now time to find a house physician post for the second six months of my pre-registration year. I had clearly not shone in my medical attachments in Oxford as no one had suggested that they would give me a post. I looked in the British Medical Journal and there was a post advertised at a University of Southampton hospital. It was advertised as a post in general medicine with an interest in respiratory medicine which I thought would be ideal for a prospective surgeon. I went down for an interview, looked around the hospital, and met the consultant in charge before the interview. It turned out that the post was 95% respiratory medicine, with a very minor interest in general medicine. Excellent for a prospective anaesthetist but less ideal for a surgeon. I discussed this and my career to date with the consultant. He said that if I wanted the post, it was mine, but he clearly realised that it was not the post that I really wanted, and with his blessing I therefore withdrew my application. The other connection that I had was with the Battle Hospital in Reading, and Mr Chesterman said that he would talk to Dr Hausmann, the senior physician at the hospital, and he would arrange for me to be offered the post. Obviously an organiser, but it may also have been that he could gain a good SHO, as Vivian might sign up for six months in Accident and Emergency with orthopaedics, And that is what happened. Rather than travelling to Reading on many days we took a married flat in the hospital and rented out our rooms in Oxford. The house was looked after very well, for the next year, by a marine sergeant major who had been one of my tenants for the previous year whilst he was working as the head of army recruitment in Oxford.

General medicine in Reading was somewhat unusually organised. Normally a team would take all of the cases on the day that they were on-call. There were slightly more medical beds at the Battle Hospital than at the Royal Berkshire Hospital and it had therefore been agreed that the general medical cases would be split in the normal way, but all of the overdoses, which averaged between two and three each day, would be taken by the Battle Hospital. This meant that we were on-call every day for some patients. As well as the normal ward beds, we also had a small coronary care unit. The team consisted of Dr Walter Hausman and Dr Andrew Pay as the consultants, a registrar and two housemen. Dr Hausman was an Austrian who had qualified from Vienna in 1935 and left Austria very soon afterwards to escape the Nazi threat. He had done some important medical research and eventually became a recognised consultant physician. Dr Pay was much younger and appeared to have a relationship with Dr Hausman where although he was a consultant, he appeared to be always a junior doctor. They both had problems. Dr Hausman had severe Parkinson's disease which made his writing extremely difficult to interpret. As I was to discover, he was a superb physician, but partly because of his Parkinson's he found it difficult to talk to the patients. We solved this one very simply by the junior doctor doing a further ward round after Dr Hausman had left and explaining everything to the patients. Dr Pay was an inveterate and very severe smoker. Halfway through a ward round he would always say that he needed a cup of tea. At least we had a cup of tea while he would have two or three cigarettes. Not long after I left, and still a young person, he died of a heart attack on a ward round.

The nursing, particularly the sister on the coronary care unit, was excellent and the unit worked very well together. I learned rapidly, and very soon the coronary care unit was left in my care over the night-time. Some of the more severe cardiac patients needed an internal catheter inserting, and when they discovered my interest in surgery that job rapidly became mine. I also learned about the psychiatric problems of the patients who were overdosing. Very clearly the vast majority had no intention of committing suicide but needed help. Our job was to keep them alive and talk to them before arranging an appointment with a psychiatrist. This was normally fairly simple but occasionally one psychiatrist in particular could be difficult. I remember a young girl who had taken a large number of aspirin tablets, had then sliced her wrist, and was only prevented from jumping out of an upstairs window by her boyfriend restraining her. All three were obviously severe attempts at suicide and the particular consultant psychiatrist tried to tell me they were not serious, and he would not come to see her. I told him that I would write the problems in the notes and say that he had refused an appointment. At that point he changed his mind and when I told Dr Hausman what had happened the following day, he totally backed me. Another patient that I remember was admitted to the coronary unit with a moderately severe heart attack. He survived and went home some two weeks later. He was the owner of a large chocolate company and a large box of chocolates appeared every day on the unit for the next three months, and even when our weights increased we were still very grateful to him.

It was not a busy job, and as Vivian was working in the casualty department I would often go along to keep her company. The nurses of course knew me from the previous three months that I had worked there, and on occasions would ask me to suture the face of a young patient. I do remember one patient who had been involved in a serious motor accident and was in a very serious condition and going rapidly blue. The casualty officer who was looking after him was clearly inexperienced and was spending his time doing an electrocardiogram. Apparently he had been told off for not doing one on a previous patient who needed one, and he did not want to make the same mistake twice. Whilst he was doing the ECG I put a chest drain in on one side, and then realised the other side also had a pneumothorax and added a second chest drain. A life that I definitely saved.

We made friends with other junior doctors and another husband and wife couple, Drs David and Val Howes, with whom we are still friendly and have holidayed with on several occasions. The six months went rapidly, and towards the end of the time Dr Hausman asked me if I would wish to apply for his registrar job. I was very flattered, but I had the problem that I was already 10 years older than my peer group, and with considerable sadness I decided not to apply, as it would have been a very helpful training post for a future surgeon.

In the 1970s when one job finished it was up to each individual to organise their next job by an application, and normally an interview. As I said earlier, I had already been offered two senior house officer posts, in plastic surgery and in the Accident Service, both at Oxford. However during my elective in Zululand, I had agreed with the Doctors Barker that I would return for six months when I had fully registered. Oxford were very happy to put off my two posts and Vivian and I started the organisation of registering in South Africa and for me to return, and for her to travel to South Africa for the first time. A few weeks later we had a nasty shock when Anthony Barker told us that our work permits for South Africa had been refused. We found out subsequently that the problem occurred when he was on a lecture tour in the United States to raise money to build another ward. He had included a section on malnutrition in the South African homelands. According to the South African government, malnutrition did not occur in the homelands, and hence the refusal. We had already bought our airline tickets which were not refundable, and then had to find other work for the six months. We sent off a series of letters, and within four days the government of Lesotho telephoned and offered both of us jobs for as long as we wished. I think now that neither of us had heard of the country, but after a little reading we accepted.

The forms for my full registration were completed and submitted, and the date on which I expected this to be completed was the date of the start of our posts in Lesotho.

TEN

SOUTHERN AFRICA

LESOTHO

Vivian and I had now been married for 18 months. She had qualified five years before me, and had also taken the Diploma in Child Health and the Diploma in Obstetrics and Gynaecology and was fully trained as a GP working for the Membership of The Royal College of General Practitioners. With that selection she was far better qualified than I was, and would instantly be useful in Lesotho.

We travelled via Johannesburg and nearly had a disaster. We were due to fly to Maseru, the capital of Lesotho but were given boarding tickets for Mauritius. Just before getting on the plane we realised the mistake – by which time the daily flight to Maseru had departed. We therefore hired a car and set off. As we were leaving Johannesburg we were flagged down, and told by the driver from the hire company that they had made a mistake as they did not have a depot in Maseru. Not in the best of temper I told them that we had to be there that day, and after some discussion it was agreed that we would leave the car nearby in Ladybrand in the Orange Free State, and a driver would take us to Maseru.

And so to Maseru. We were interviewed by the Director of the Health Service, Dr Moshoeshoe who told us that we would have a formal appointment interview later. He then asked us what our interests were. I said surgery, at which he smiled and said, "The second surgeon to the country went on holiday yesterday, and you can do his job until he returns." The day

I registered I was second surgeon to a million people, and if that is not rapid promotion, what is?

We were put up in the local hotel and given a tour of the hospital where I met Dr Siddique. He was originally from Pakistan and had done some training in England where he had passed the Fellowship of the Royal College, and had then got stuck as an SHO in, I think, Barnsley in Yorkshire. He had then migrated to Lesotho where he had been working for some years. He was a delightful colleague and a capable surgeon. Incredibly I met his son, a doctor, in London forty years later when we were both on medical duty at Wimbledon.

The plan was for us to work in Maseru for two weeks whilst they made sure that we could do Caesarean sections, which were a constant need in the country, before sending us to a hospital in another town. Because of Vivian's six month job in obstetrics and gynaecology, and my experience in Zululand we both had some experience. My two weeks of surgery were interesting. Dr Siddique and I would do a ward round and decide who definitely needed an operation. He would say that he had done the operation needed, I would say that I had assisted at the relevant operation, he would say that he had seen the operation, and I would say that I had read about it – and the operating list was divided up between us. One problem, as so often in developing countries, was the problem of anaesthetics. In Maseru there was an English junior doctor who had passed the Diploma in Anaesthetics (DA) which was the most basic British qualification – and which ceased to exist in the 1970s. His job in Maseru was to keep two patients asleep in the two operating theatres with the help of two medical assistants. He would run between the theatres with a very worried look on his face. It was an interesting two weeks, made somewhat difficult by the complete absence of a surgical textbook. Because of the aircraft weight limit I had taken only one textbook to study for the Primary FRCS examination, and a physiology book is not of much use in the operating theatre to a surgeon.

There was a surprisingly active social life both in the hospital and in the city. We played tennis, went on natural history walks, and borrowed books from the British Council library. We were also invited to the house of a doctor in the hospital whose wife had a garden full of injured animals that she was looking after. Not everyone has patted a lammergeier (a bearded vulture) on the head which is well above waist level. A fascinating afternoon and an excellent meal.

Our next posting was to Teyateyaneng, known locally as TY, where we took over the hospital and the house of a Canadian doctor and his wife. They were members of the Bahai faith of which we knew nothing. Apparently all members had to work for two years either preaching or working in problem communities, which is what they were doing. As well as the house I was delighted to discover that he had a medical library which I used for the two weeks that we were there. The most difficult part of the job was dealing with psychiatric patients. These are a problem at any time, and the problem is severely exacerbated when there is a total language barrier. We did find that there is in Southern Africa a much greater acceptance of psychiatric patients who live in their local village much more often than happens in the United Kingdom.

Our last posting in Lesotho was to Leribe, the second city to the north-west, and one and a half hours away at the end of what was then the only tarred road in the country. Technically the town is called Hlotse, in the district of Leribe, but to confuse everybody it was generally called Leribe. There we joined a Dutch doctor, Dr Fritz Pasma who was on a year's contract. He had been there for some time on his own and was delighted when we arrived. The hospital (Photo 10.1) was nearly twice as large as TY and very busy. As well as the normal patients we also had to do medicals on local people wishing to work in the South African gold mines. We were told by one of our medical assistants that previous North Korean doctors would go down the line of 30 people 'listening' to their chests with the earpieces of the stethoscope around the neck and not in their ears. Certainly a faster way of doing it. When examining for physical disability I devised a gymnastics class with all the recruits copying what I was doing at the same time. It was easy to pick up anybody who was struggling. The miners working away caused another problem. They would come home to their wives for two weeks every year and a few weeks afterwards there were a number of ladies coming to the out-patients with Total Body Pain. Vivian worked out that this meant – am I pregnant? And if not, why not? One of the causes was venereal disease (VD) which was brought back from the mines by the men, and we all rapidly became experts at recognising and treating it. We had

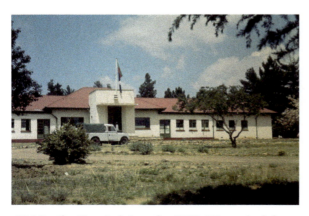

10.1 Leribe Hospital. Lesotho 1973. We worked there for two months in 1973,

an American doctor for a short visit talking about VD and he was teaching that gay sex did not happen in Lesotho. From our observation of the position of some of the VD lesions we knew that he was talking rubbish, and told him so. His response was that local people had told him that homosexuality did not exist in the country – and he had believed it. Another connected problem was that the whole of the country ran out of penicillin which was the standard treatment of VD, because it had not been ordered. We had also run out of Plaster of Paris for fixing fractures and even Elastoplast. We sent a driver to the stores in Maseru and four hours later he came back with one roll of Elastoplast. Vivian was then persuaded to visit the stores which was full of the many things that we needed. The storeman thought that his job was keeping the store full rather than distributing the goods. Vivian disabused him and came back with the Land Rover full, and probably enough of many things to last the Leribe Hospital for several years.

Other problems that we came across included the lack of an X-Ray machine and the inability to do simple laboratory work. Our medical assistants showed us an X-Ray machine and a basic laboratory which were still in their original packages where they had been put when they had been donated to the country. Fritz's partner put together the laboratory and she then started doing basic tests. I put together the X-Ray machine and from first principles worked out how to take radiographs. There was also a problem when a blood transfusion was required. We kept only two units of blood, and only of the commonest blood group which was A+. This was carried by 90+% of the Lesotho population. If more blood was needed it took several hours to have it sent from Maseru. There had been a national shortage which was, and still is, common in many countries. Almost the only guaranteed source was within a family. This had been partially solved in Lesotho by offering nearly all prisoners two weeks off their sentence every six months for donating a unit of blood. Everybody gained from the idea. The prisoner thought that he had earned his remission. The state saved money, and the medical service had sufficient blood. The only problem which arose later was the incidence of positive HIV amongst the prisoners, and I have not discovered how this has been solved.

As I said earlier a very common problem in developing countries is anaesthesia, as medically qualified anaesthetists were, and are, uncommon and the anaesthetics is often done by medical assistants. In Leribe this was of a poor, and almost dangerous level, particularly for caesarean sections and we were told that before the three of us arrived there had been several deaths. To improve the situation somewhat I took over the anaesthetics. For the caesarean operations I used the local anaesthetic method devised by the Barkers in Zululand. For general anaesthetics I would put the patient to sleep, and either Vivian or Fritz would keep them asleep whilst I operated, and I would then wake them up. There were EMO machines using ether and oxygen (Chapter 6) but as the initial effect was for some patients to become very restless and need holding down, this could be a problem with large men. There was in Leribe a halothane plug-on addition which was used at the beginning of the anaesthetic, and which much more rapidly settled the patient – when halothane was available. There are other problems of ether anaesthetics. Firstly cautery cannot be used as ether is extremely flammable and an explosion would occur, and secondly it can take a long time for the patient to wake up after the surgery. One of the first patients that I anaesthetised and operated on was extremely ill before the operation, and the sister on the ward said,

"His time has come." This was a very common statement in Southern Africa when no hope was thought to exist either within the family or the medical staff. For that particular patient I did not accept this and the only way of giving him suitable post-operative care was for me to do it. I was awake with him for most of the night, and after his survival the sister began to believe me.

A laryngoscope is the instrument that is used for putting a tube into the airway, and there were three laryngoscopes available in Leribe Hospital but no tubes. This tragically caused one unnecessary death which I still regret. A man had been stabbed in the abdomen three days previously and when he came to the hospital he had a severe problem with internal bleeding. The only option was an operation. This was going well until he vomited, and without a tube the vomit went into his lungs, and he died on the table. This was very upsetting for his family and for us, and also for the person who had stabbed him as the case became one of murder. I have always felt that this was unfair as the fault was with the Government for the lack of equipment. I asked Maseru for some tubes and they said that they had no spares. I therefore drove across the border to the nearest large hospital in South Africa and borrowed a set of tubes of the relevant sizes. They happily acknowledged that this would entail a new definition of the word 'borrowed'.

We discovered that our North Korean predecessors had cancelled an out-patient clinic in a small village in the mountains about five or six miles east of Leribe, and our local contacts told us that there was a hope that we could re-establish this. I took the hospital Land Rover and a medical assistant as

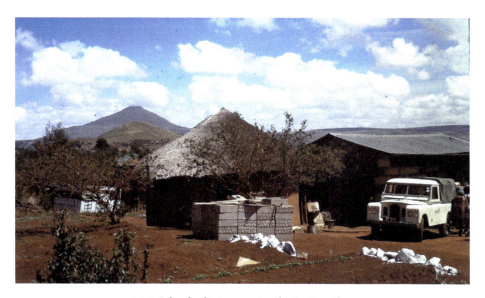

10.2 A bush clinic near Leribe in Lesotho.

guide and translator and drove to the village (Photo 10.2). An interesting drive that took almost an hour, and almost totally in low-range. We then had an indaba (actually a Zulu or Xhosa word commonly used rather than the Sotho equivalent). The head man and all the village males sat in a circle with us, and the ladies all stood around in a wider circle, but did not speak. The discussion went on for about two hours and we agreed that we would do a fortnightly clinic whenever we had the staff and the 'road' was passable. I remember at a later clinic a patient being brought in by wheelbarrow! In the open back of the Land Rover there was a mattress and one or possibly two people could be transported back to the hospital, but not in any comfort at all.

When the equipment and stores had been sorted the work between the three of us went well for the two months.

There were other problems. We had been allocated a very pleasant bungalow in grounds of about two acres, and it even had separate staff quarters. In the morning of our first night Vivian knowing that I was collecting butterflies and bugs discovered several bugs in the bed. From my Zambian experience I recognised them instantly as bed-bugs, and looking at Vivian noticed a straight line of bites to which she had reacted quite markedly. Luckily I did not react.

We phoned Maseru and asked what they were going to do. They said that they must have been introduced by the North Koreans who had been in the house, and they had wondered why they had kept ordering DDT. Clearly the bed-bugs were resistant to DDT. We moved into a very pleasant local hotel whilst the house was fumigated and also repainted as they were indeed very resistant bugs. When we moved back into the house there were a continual row of people knocking on the door asking for employment, and we eventually gave in and employed Grace, a lovely elderly lady who looked after us superbly and also told any further callers that she was definitely in post. Some weeks later she told us that she wished that the British were still in charge, as the country had worked much better. After a couple of weeks one of the ward nurses asked if she could rent our staff hut for her, her husband and daughter. Clearly it was not ours to rent, but we allowed them to move in, and it increased our security. The only thing that I regret about the house and the garden was that at the time I was not a bird ringer, and the most marvellous site full of birds went to waste.

There was a social life of the town based on a club where tennis was clearly important. We were surprised at the high average level of those playing, and we had some excellent games. There we met another Englishman who had been seconded by the British police to work as deputy head of the Lesotho police. He invited me to go with him in the police Land Rover across Lesotho. Vivian and Fritz agreed to stand in for the necessary two days and the two of us with a driver set off on a journey that I have not forgotten. In 1973 the whole journey was on a dirt track. The common form of transport was the horse, and these were everywhere. We did not see another vehicle for the 148 miles to the top of the Sani pass which took nine hours (Photo 10.3). At one point we forded a fast flowing river and were not cheered by the driver telling us that a vehicle had been swept sideways off the road and the occupants killed only two weeks previously. To my amazement we arrived at our overnight accommodation which was a ski lodge – the only one then in Southern Africa. Although close to mid summer at 9,500ft above sea level it was still cold. The next day was the trip down the pass. Again a dirt track, with an average gradient of 1 in 3 and considerably steeper in places, and we were in low range with three point turns on most of the corners. Interesting. The journey back was on a real road in South Africa and only took about four hours.

Whilst we were in Lesotho. Vivian and I bought an inexpensive VW camper van in South Africa for our future planned travels. In this we visited two other hospitals. One was a Seventh Day Adventist mission hospital specialising in eye surgery. Unfortunately we went on a Saturday without knowing that this was their sabbath. Although welcomed we did not see the hospital working. The

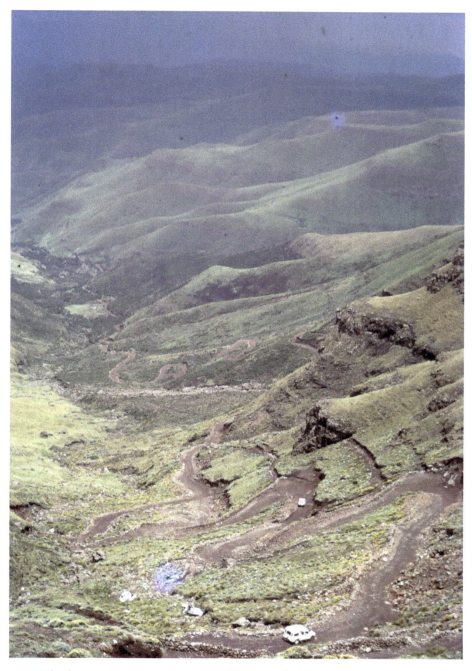
10.3 The famous Sani Pass joining Lesotho to South Africa in the north-east of the country.

other hospital was a Swiss ecumenical mission hospital in, I think, Mafeteng where we were welcomed by a lady doctor who had worked there on her own for several years. A third proposed visit was to St James's Catholic Mission Hospital which was in the mountains in the middle of the country. This was to be for a weekend, but the wet weather finished this idea as the VW slowly slid into a ditch where we spent the night (Photo 10.4). Luckily the next day the rain had stopped, and I was able to extract the van and we arrived home with no further problem.

I think it was in Lesotho that the attitude of Southern Africans to death became clear. 'His time has come' was a common statement by family and by medical staff and it often took a considerable effort by us for them to agree that 'perhaps his time has not come'. This attitude by a family did mean that the doctors were not to blame when a relative died, and what a complete contrast this was to many other countries around the world. Another problem in Lesotho was that it was a Roman Catholic country, and therefore contraception was banned. The only way to stop constant pregnancies was a 'child spacing programme' which happened if a baby was breast fed for two years. A problem that was occurring was an acceptance that artificial milk must be better as it was used by white South Africans. Vivian and Fritz, who were covering the obstetrics did their best to counteract this.

We much enjoyed our three months, but just before we left we were summoned to our appointment interview with the Minister of Health and the two senior medical doctors in Maseru. Slightly weird we thought, but the reason for the interview

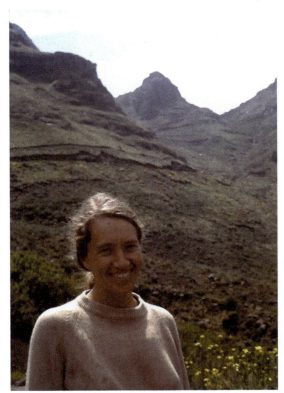

10.4 Travels in Lesotho. A very mountainous country. My wife Vivian.

became clear as the whole interview was asking us both to stay for longer. We were luckily able to say, quite truthfully, that we were already committed elsewhere.

We left Fritz and his partner on their own, and heard later that Fritz had had to do twenty post-mortems on Christmas day after some local fighting.

ZULULAND AND SOUTH AFRICA

On the 15th of December we drove through the Transkei and across Zululand (now KwaZulu-Natal) to the Charles Johnson Memorial Hospital, to be greeted by the Doctors Barker and shown to our rondavel in which to recover. I had spent three months of my student elective there. Although only two and a half years earlier the hospital had changed somewhat. The doctors were still a mixture of British and South African. The nursing school was still vibrant, but the medical students had changed in that there were no British students, and as I was to discover very soon most of the South African students had some psychological problems. Clearly the Barkers had developed a reputation for helping such students, and I am certain that it was deserved. Certainly they would not have turned such students away, although it probably reduced the standards to some extent.

The next morning Anthony told us that the Government, having refused our work permits for 1973, had now granted them for 1974. This was of no use to us as we had already planned to tour Southern Africa for the next three months and then I had my job in Oxford on our return. We therefore worked illegally at Nqutu for two weeks. My outstanding memory of those two weeks was an evening walking across the bush with the nurses by the light of the candles that they were carrying, and listening to them carol singing. Knowing where we were going on our tour Anthony suggested that we contact Dr Merriweather in the Scottish Mission Hospital at Molepolole in Botswana, and go with him to visit the clinic in the desert that he did every month to treat bushmen (San people). This was arranged for about for four weeks time. Having had a Christmas and New Year amongst friends we drove away on the 1st of January. It had been touch and go. This was at the time of the oil embargo and strict fuel rationing. At the last minute, tourists were allowed extra fuel, but only on certain days of the week. Carefully planned journeys became imperative, and extra fuel in cans was banned. The other problem was that the speed limits on the main raids had been reduced to 80kph (50 mph), and cars were being timed between towns. A very heavy fine was levied if excess average speed occurred. In our old VW this did not worry us as the top speed was not much above 50mph.

Our tour started by driving to Durban and then down the coast to stay with the same farming family who had put me up when I was hitch hiking on my previous visit three years earlier. We then travelled through the Transkei where we stopped for one night by a small pond and were kept awake all night by dozens of very noisy frogs. In East London we joined the famous Garden Route which we followed to Cape Town. We had two days in Cape Town, and as there was both a long queue for the cable car for Table Mountain, and to save both time and money we walked to the top. It was a fairly hard walk, but not at all dangerous.

The next morning we started the two days drive to Molepolole. On arrival a Scottish sister came out to meet us, and having discovered that we were doctors asked me if I would quickly come and help the local doctor finish a Caesarean as he was having serious trouble. When the operation was finished, she found out who we were, and why we had arrived there. Having told her that it had been arranged with Dr Merriweather, we learnt the terrible news that he had been involved in a car crash two days earlier. His wife and one daughter had been killed, and he, and another daughter were seriously injured and in hospital. It was beginning to get dark, and we therefore camped in the car park overnight. Another more experienced local doctor came the next morning, and as there was nothing else useful that we could do we set off towards Windhoek in what was then South West Africa (now Namibia). The Rev Dr Alfred Merriweather survived, and many years later after he had retired, we met him and his second wife on a return visit to Botswana. A remarkable man who had done an enormous amount for Botswana including being the first Speaker of the House when the country had become independent. He was also the personal physician to the President. Botswana is now a very different country after the discovery of diamonds in enormous quantities, but when we were there in 1974 there were about 8 miles of tarred road in total. Driving along a dirt road one day we were following an enormous dust trail. When we eventually caught up we discovered a tractor dragging a tree behind it. Certainly a novel way of grading a road, as obviously the country could not afford a proper grader. There was no hurry and we drove slowly, not that there was any other way to do it with the condition of the roads, to the Fish River

Canyon. This was an incredible drive through desert and neither of us had previously seen such a landscape. And then in the middle of nowhere with no vegetation in sight we would come across animals. There was also some excellent birdwatching. In particular one noted the birds of prey, and then in a single kokerboom tree there would be thousands of nests of sociable weavers.

South West Africa had been a German colony until 1915, and many of the residents, especially in Luderitz in the south, spoke only German, and shopping would have been difficult had Vivian not spoken German fluently. Many of the tall Herero women in their magnificent long dresses left over from a century before were very elegant and again their second language was German and not English or Afrikaans. Our original plan had been to visit the famous Etosha nature reserve, but our timing was amiss, and it was closed for two months for the breeding season of the animals. We therefore drove slowly up the coast observing the seabirds, the flamingos and the multitudinous seals to Walvis Bay and camped each night. Walvis Bay was then an isolated part of South Africa. We went a little further north where there was some vegetation which was watered not by rain, but by severe mists each morning. The next part of the trip was to the capital Windhoek. This was architecturally a typical colonial town with almost no building more than two stories. My main memory of Windhoek was a magnificent sewage works – certainly magnificent for the bird life there.

After about five weeks of travelling we were becoming a little bored, and although our original plan had been for two and a half months we decided to look for a month's work. I remembered enjoying my previous two weeks in Rhodesia and contacted them. There was an immediate response of welcome and two posts were offered. We therefore set off back through the Kalahari game reserve in Botswana and nearly had another disaster. The main road through the reserve towards Rhodesia was the bed of the river. We were gently progressing along this. At one point we had stopped for our lunch and were sitting in the back of the camper with the doors open, I was taking a cine film of a nearby lion which had clearly smelt the food. When it started licking its lips, the doors were rapidly closed and we set off. A few hours later there was an unbelievable thunderstorm and the road rapidly turned into a river. Our only option was to attempt to drive across the desert on a compass bearing. We succeeded and very nearly got stuck twice. There in the middle of the desert appeared some young lads who for ten cents each, pushed us out. What they were doing in the desert we never did discover. We crossed the border illegally as night fell, camped and found a border post the next day. We discovered afterwards that we were probably the only two wheel drive vehicle to get out for two weeks, and that the storm had been the first rain for eight years.

RHODESIA

After a brief meeting in Salisbury (now Harare) with the Department of Health we discovered that we were to work in Marendellas (now Marondera) in the north east of the country. We arrived and met an elderly Irish doctor, Dr Duncan, who had been there for many years. It was a rather large hospital for one doctor, and the reason came out fairly rapidly. There had been an Italian 'doctor' who turned out not to be a doctor at all. One of the local Shona medical assistants had had the courage to report him for repairing a hernia by cutting only the skin and then sewing it up. The truth then came out that he had been an operating assistant in Italy, had forged his certificates and moved to Rhodesia to earn more money and become a 'doctor'. He had left in a hurry a few weeks previously.

Although being ruled by Ian Smith under UDI (Unilateral Declaration of Independence) there was no apartheid and the hospital therefore took people of all races. There was an excellent matron, and the nursing staff were predominantly white and the medical assistants all Shona. The Shona were the majority tribe in the country, and the language, which is the national language, is spoken by 70% of the population. The Ndebele live in the south west and the language, closely related to Zulu, is spoken by 20% of the population. In 1974 Rhodesia (now Zimbabwe) was a rich and happy country, and was known as the bread basket of Southern Africa for its farming exports. How life changes.

We settled into the flat that we were given and started work. Most of my work was in the operating theatres, and for once there were no problems with anaesthesia. The medical assistant was an absolute natural. However difficult the case he just carried on with no complaints and with total success. If the patient needed an endotracheal tube or mechanical ventilation, although there was no respirator, he would compress the bag manually for as long as was needed. A remarkable feat.

There were problems on occasions. On one day there was a lady in theatre with a problem with twins which turned out be locked twins. I was anaesthetising her, and Vivian was attempting the delivery when she suddenly,

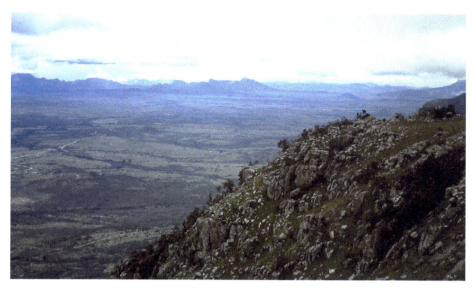

10.5 Rhodesia. From the top of the Nyanga mountains to the north-east of the country.

and for the first time in her life fainted. Our senior colleague Dr Duncan took over the delivery. Afterwards Matron put Vivian on a diet of meat to strengthen her up, but that made her somewhat nauseated. When we returned to England one week later, a pregnancy test diagnosed the problem.

We spent a weekend in the Nyanga mountains (Photo 10.5). We had been well paid. The final problem was getting our money back to England. Direct transfers were not allowed under the UDI rules, but luckily we still had a bank account in Lesotho. In two steps our money was transferred. For the first time in my life we made a profit from a bank, and I still do not know how.

The six months in Southern Africa were an incredible experience and gave us both an enormous benefit, both to our medical knowledge and even the experience of running a hospital. I am sure that the entry on my CV made my applications for jobs more successful. I had done something different. Ever since I have recommended to junior doctors to follow our example, and when short listing or interviewing I am always looking for something unusual on their CV.

The six weeks of touring away from medicine were also my longest time for fifty years until the pandemic of 2020, which limited my life considerably.

ELEVEN

SENIOR HOUSE OFFICER AND REGISTRAR

THE TRAINING SYSTEM IN THE 1970s

The training of consultants in all specialties in the 1970s would not now in 2022 be recognised, and hence a brief summary may be useful.

After the satisfactory conclusion of a minimum of a year in house jobs then one could become fully registered with the General Medical Council. A decision had to be made concerning one's future career. Did one want to be a hospital doctor, a general practitioner or to do any other form of work, for instance being a missionary doctor or working in the pharmaceutical industry? If one of the latter two, one could work completely independently. No further training, qualifications or assessments would be needed for the remainder of one's life. Training to become a GP had been discussed and trialled for many years, but it was not until 1976 that it became necessary to do a formal three year training before one could become a full partner in a general practice.

In hospital practice it had for many years been necessary to do a succession of training posts going up through the stages of Senior House Officer (SHO), Registrar (Reg) and Senior Registrar (SR) before reaching clinical independence as a Consultant. In all hospital posts up to consultant the person was known as a junior doctor, and this was independent of age or experience.

SHO posts normally lasted for six months and two to four such posts were expected. They could be appointed either with or without an interview. Reg posts were normally for two years, with an assessment after one year. These posts required an advertisement and a formal interview. One or two such posts were normal. The SR post was normally for two years, but could be prolonged for as long as necessary if the performance was satisfactory and a reasonable, but unspecified, number of consultant job applications were made.

During these years the relevant specialist higher qualification exams had to be taken and passed. In surgery these were the Primary and Final Examinations of one of the Royal Colleges of Surgeons. The four colleges were (and are) of England, of Glasgow, of Edinburgh or of Ireland. In theory these were of equal merit – but no one quite believed that. In medicine the examinations were Part 1 and then the final examination of one of the Royal Colleges of Physicians. The other main specialties had similar systems. Because of the popularity, and of the number of people wanting to specialise in the different subjects, the competitive levels were very different. Then, but certainly not now, anaesthetics was the specialty with an easier route to a consultant post. It was said that if the candidate could write their name, they were appointed as a registrar, and if they could do it in joined up writing, then a senior registrar post was theirs. Plastic surgery, followed by neurosurgery and then general surgery were, and are, the most competitive surgical specialities.

This system had one very major advantage. If someone was not making the expected level at any grade, then they were not promoted to the next grade within that specialty. What was missing then was a mentoring system for juniors going up through the ranks, and it was normally left for a person to realise that they were either not being shortlisted for interviews, or failing in the interviews. They could then stay in a grade, become an associate specialist, or change subject. The associate specialist posts were also used by those failing to obtain the necessary qualifications, by those wishing to work part time, or overseas doctors without the examinations or the CV enhancements that were necessary.

The successful trainees then applied for and could be appointed to a consultant post. Unless ill health intervened, this was a permanent post until retirement age, which was then 65 for all specialties except psychiatry, when it was 60. It was possible for a consultant to be suspended or dismissed for clinical incompetence or for misdemeanours, but those were then rare cases.

OXFORD – THE ACCIDENT SERVICE

In October 1974 I returned to Oxford to my previously arranged posting in the Accident Service. The Accident Service then was almost certainly unique. It was truly an accident service. The reception desk was ordered to only register a patient if they had had an accident within twenty-four hours, or if their general practitioner was outside the Oxford area, or if the patient was not registered with a GP at all. If the patient coming in had a medical problem they were handed over to the medical team on call in an adjacent area; after urgent resuscitation by the accident service if that was necessary.

There were often complaints from patients that they could not make an appointment with their GP. Which actually meant that they had not tried, as the GPs all knew the system. In these patients an appointment with the GP was made by the receptionist. There was one local GP who objected, and she was eventually struck off by the General Medical Council for this and for several other valid reasons.

The service was medically staffed by five SHOs, two surgical registrars, one neurosurgical registrar, one senior registrar and an orthopaedic consultant. The last job was shared by five consultants on a daily rotation.

The SHOs were appointed to start on a monthly basis which had the enormous advantage that there was a spread of experience at all times. For our first two months we were primarily on the wards looking after the patients and operating or assisting in theatres. That part of the post was on a one in two on-call rota. The final four months we were on the 'front door', seeing and treating when relevant all the patients as they came in, or referring them to one of the registrars. This was extremely busy, and we were on a two in three rota. Without a doubt it was the most exhausting period of my career, especially as I was studying for the Primary examination for the Fellowship of the Royal College of Surgeons at the same time, and also starting a research project.

Anyone now working in A and E departments would not recognise the above workload. Firstly the patient load has completely changed. In 1996 GPs ceased to do 24 hour care of their own patients, and this has meant an enormous increase in the number of patients attending accident departments despite an on-call service being arranged. I, and many older doctors, are convinced that this was one of the greatest disasters in patient care in the United Kingdom for generations. Secondly all patients who walk in the door are now automatically seen in A and E departments, and there is a government requirement that they should either be discharged or admitted within a four hour time limit from their registration. This can mean that if there is a delay in laboratory testing or in an Xray department, to fiddle the system the patient is quite unjustifiably admitted. Thirdly no one now would believe that we ran the A and E department in a major teaching hospital with one orthopaedic consultant on call. Mr John Cockin, a full time orthopaedic hand surgeon, oversaw the department as an additional duty, with only nine junior doctors. Mr Cockin was famous for having a notice outside his outpatient clinic saying 'Cockin Hand Clinic', and to the delight of all the medical students refused to remove it when the removal was suggested by the management.

A recent count (2020) at the John Radcliffe Hospital showed 25 consultants with five additional military senior doctors staffing the present unit. Another problem is that all of the SHO posts start at the beginning of either August or February and there is no breadth of experience in each intake. It is known that there is a higher problem rate in treatment and outcomes during the first weeks of these months. But perhaps they get some sleep nowadays.

In 1974 the accident service consisted of a waiting room with receptionists and an open plan examination room with a large desk with a doctor at each end of one side. There were four cubicles for the more severely injured patients or for discrete examinations. Two of the cubicles were very sensibly soundproofed for examining children and babies. Finally there was a small minor operating theatre. The adjacent medical area was a small ward, and on the wall there was a plaque saying; 'A patient in this bed was the first in the world to receive penicillin'.

For those who needed admission there was Cronshaw Ward for men. This was mostly occupied by young men with fractured femurs (thigh bones), and in the days before internal fixation they would be in-patients for eight to ten weeks with their legs strung up on a frame attached to a special bed. Beside this was Cronshaw Annexe, a small intensive care ward for serious head injuries who did not need surgery. On the opposite side of the main corridor was Victoria Ward for ladies. This was mainly filled with elderly ladies with fractured necks of the femur. Surgery for this injury was just beginning and their stay was less prolonged. And very often all three of our wards would be filled, and we would have extra patients boarded out anywhere else in the hospital. To the best of my knowledge no patient was ever refused admission or sent to another hospital except for burns and spinal injuries when they were transferred to Stoke Mandeville Hospital.

My first two months were admitting and looking after these in-patients which could number one hundred. There are always amusing stories about accident wards. Late one night there was a very belligerent patient on Cronshaw Ward and I had been called to give him an injection to calm him down. As I walked on to the ward one of the other patients who worked for British Leyland looked at me and said,

"What are you doing here – you were on the day shift." I politely told him about our 32 hour on call shifts. I have two memories from Cronshaw Annexe. The first was a young lass of about fifteen whose memory was slowly returning after some days following a head injury. On one of my visits her father said that he had not realised that she had injured her chest as well as her head. I was somewhat baffled as she had not injured her chest, and so I asked him why he thought that had happened. He said, "There is quite marked bruising". With some embarrassment, I had to explain that to assess her level of consciousness a gentle pressure was exerted on the sternum to evaluate the patient's reaction. Clearly she either bruised very easily, or one of us, or a nurse, had been somewhat over-exuberant in our assessments. Her father took it very well.

The second patient, Michael, was a twenty year old man who was recovering from a severe head injury, but was clearly 'still away with the fairies'. This is not uncommon as the conscious level improves but normally lasts for a few hours or a day. Michael was not settling at all after several days. The marvellous sister worked out that he had been a drug addict, and one of his friends was feeding him LSD – on an intensive care ward! Sister then asked me to arrange a psychiatrist to visit Michael. I did this and told sister that a very pleasant and remarkably normal psychiatrist, Dr Gaff would be coming the following day. When I next went onto the ward a not very happy sister said,

"I thought you said that the psychiatrist would be normal – he was a complete lunatic."

"You can't mean Dr Gaff surely?" was my response.

"That was not his name," she said. "It was something double barrelled."

It must have been Dr Seymour Spencer to whom the request must have been passed, and how correct was her diagnosis. He was well known at the beginning of a consultation to instruct new patients to wake him up if he went to sleep. Although very different he was very much liked by his patients.

For one of my two months on the ward I was with Peter Teddy. On Victoria ward was a lovely old time sister, Mary Hastings, who had run it for many years, and was not too keen on change. As I said the ward was almost completely occupied by old ladies with fractured necks of femur. Being old they normally came in with a variety of other diagnoses and on various pills. One of our first jobs was to prescribe the pills that they had been on, and it dawned on Peter and me that half of the pills were treating the complications caused by the other half. After our teaching from Dr Wollner, the senior geriatrician, we had a good look at the diagnoses and the treatments and decided that on average about 80% of the medication could be stopped, and in the well monitored space of the ward, if a problem recurred, the treatment could be restarted. This worked extremely well and many of the patients went home with far fewer pills, and with less possible complications. The next thing Peter and I did was to look at the sleeping pills given to all the patients. There is the famous answer given in a nursing examination. 'The first duty of the night sister is to wake up all the patients and give them their sleeping tablets'. And certainly we noticed that when we were called in the middle of the night that many of the patients would be confused, often shouting, or far worse with their healing fractures, trying to get out of bed. We therefore decided to ban all sleeping tablets, and did we have a fight with the nurses and with Sister Hastings! But we fought back, and amazingly after about two weeks Sister thanked us and said that the report was that the ward had never been so quiet during the night. Sister Hastings became a good friend for the rest of our time in the unit.

During the first two months we also covered the acute neurosurgical admissions. Having spent several weeks and many weekends as a student locum on the neurosurgical unit this held few fears for me. By far the commonest patients had minor head injuries – partly undergraduates playing sport and partly from car accidents as they were then known (now Road Traffic Incidents – RTI's). Mr John Potter's rule was that anyone who had had a period of loss of consciousness was admitted for monitoring for twenty-four hours to make certain that no deteriorating injury was missed, and also to emphasise, both to us and to the patient, the potential seriousness of a head injury. The first week of the autumn term when undergraduates were trying to impress with their rugby skills was particularly busy.

The saddest of all of the patients that I looked after was a Royal Navy Captain who on exercises in the Far East had had an epileptic fit. The Oxford unit was first on call for all of the Services neurological and neurosurgical cases, and he was brought to us with remarkable speed. When he arrived, he was over the fits, but despite multiple investigations, no cause was found for the cause of the problem. The tragedy was that a man who was possibly the youngest Captain in the Royal Navy at the time could no longer be given the responsibility of commanding at sea, and his career was finished.

Another very sad patient was a fourteen year old boy with a brain tumour who was coming to the end of his short life. He was a student at St Edward's School in Oxford and one of his last requests was to meet Douglas Bader who had also been a student at the school. I was detailed to meet Douglas Bader in the morning and introduce them to each other. Unfortunately Mr Bader was delayed until the afternoon, by which time I was in the operating theatre and I missed meeting a man who had always been one of my schoolboy heroes. Much more importantly he did meet the young lad.

After those two months life became even busier for the four months on the 'front door', and also operating in our minor theatre. The rota was two out of three nights in the hospital. The first night one was up all night, the second night in theory one was on second call, but at weekends it was normally also a full night working. Before the first on call night shift, the afternoon from lunch until 1800hrs was off, and during this time one of the new ward based SHOs would cover if required. This time off was on one occasion of major importance to me. On the 15th October my wife had been admitted to the John Radcliffe Hospital maternity unit, and during the five hours that I was off-duty she timed it perfectly and I was able to deliver my elder daughter. Clare was the last baby that I delivered by the normal way.

The two registrars alternated duties on a one in two rota, and the senior registrar and the head injury neurosurgical registrar were on call permanently, but protected to some extent by the registrars.

Those four months are now a blur in my memory. I do remember three unusual occasions. The first was when a young lad in his late teens was screaming around the unit in the middle of an LSD trip. He was grabbed by us and a couple of the medical students, the medical registrar was called to give him an intravenous injection to quieten him. He arrived and eventually found a vein. The injection went in, and one of the medical students collapsed to the floor. Wrong arm. The registrar, who was known not to be too good, never lived it down.

The second occasion was when we had just had a major road traffic accident through the door. One patient had died, and two others needed serious and urgent attention. When this had been sorted, the next patient in the queue complained bitterly that he had been waiting for an hour with no one looking after him. It was the only time in my career that I lost my temper with a patient.

The third patient was a small and very well spoken gentleman that appeared in A and E with a hand injury. He was carrying a small leather case, and when we told him that he was to be admitted he said that what was in the case was all that he needed. The story came out over the next few days. He had been a Professor within the University but unfortunately alcohol took over his life. He lost his job, and gently drank the brandy to which he was addicted. An uncle had left him sufficient money to buy two bottles a day – and that was what was in his small case. I told him that we could prescribe the brandy for him, but having tasted the NHS brandy, he decided to stay with his own. An interesting man to talk to, and especially as he was very happy with his situation and totally uninterested in looking for a cure of his alcoholism.

In 1974 only a doctor could certify death. The ambulances had a simple code as they drove into the accident service entrance. If there was a dead patient aboard, they gave a single toot of their horn, and when we had finished seeing the patient at the desk, we would go outside to certify the death. If they had a seriously injured patient the full blast of the horns was given and there was an immediate response from us. The old system led to some unusual situations. My wife Vivian, as a police surgeon, remembers two unusual cases. Somebody digging in their garden dug up a skull. This was reported to the police who called Vivian as only she could certify the death. The archaeologists were then called in to decide if it was a stone age skull. The second one was after a death on the railway. The head was separated from the body by some yards – but again only a doctor could certify that the person was dead. The law has now changed to be much more sensible and a qualified nurse or a paramedic can confirm a death.

With the encouragement of Mr Cockin I set up and, with Peter Teddy and my other colleagues, did a research trial for patients with hand lacerations comparing Triplopen, (a penicillin injection), penicillin tablets (flucloxacillin) taken by mouth for seven days, or no antibiotics. This produced the result that neither was slightly better than either antibiotic and this also saved the patient in the Triplopen group some pain, and the third who were in the flucloxacillin group from diarrhoea. It also reduced the risk of having an allergic response or of developing antibiotic resistance. What made the greatest difference to the rate of infection was keeping the dressing dry. The work was published in the British Journal of Surgery.

The six months came to an end. Never in the rest of my career had I been so grateful and so worn out. I had learnt an enormous amount, had gained confidence both in my ability to diagnose patients and in doing minor surgery.

The surgery, particularly sewing up facial injuries caused by windscreen injuries which were very common in the days before seat belts, and with my experience in plastic surgery most of them came my way. I remember one occasion which I mentioned previously of a severely injured patient with fractures of his legs and multiple facial lacerations from a windscreen injury. Mr Taylor, the orthopaedic surgeon who had been my internal examiner for my surgery finals was operating with the registrar on his legs whilst I was putting in some 300 sutures into his face. He finished before me, and then sat and watched me for about an hour whilst I finished the face. Afterwards his registrar said that he could not believe it, as Mr Taylor was known to have very little patience.

Somehow during those six months I found time to study and pass the Primary examination for the Royal College of Surgeons. As a postscript Peter Teddy, even in his schooldays, had always wanted to be a neurosurgeon and he did become a consultant neurosurgeon at Oxford. and then moved to Australia. Whilst he was at Oxford we worked together on the occasional patient from the Spinal Injury service at Stoke Mandeville.

There were quiet times and one could be on call from the local pub, the Royal Oak (Photo 11.1), as mobile phones and long distance bleeps were not then available the porters could cross the road and call the person needed. It was known to us as the Chapel. Patients could be very impressed when one asked a colleague if one could meet him in Chapel when he had finished the care of the patient.

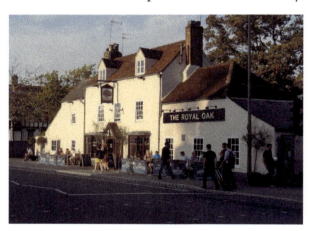

11.1 The Royal Oak pub was directly opposite the Infirmary. In the days before mobile phones and long range bleeps we socialised there even when on call as the Hospital porters could walk across and call us. It was known as 'The Chapel' which could lead to some interesting situations.

I finished my six-month appointment in the accident service in Oxford and had two months to wait for the start of the plastic surgery post. Needless to say I found another locum and during these eight weeks I did a locum registrar post in general surgery in Luton.

LUTON AND DUNSTABLE HOSPITAL

Awaiting the start of my second post at Oxford I cannot now remember if my knowledge of a vacancy for a locum was passed to me by word of mouth or by reading the vacancies section of the British Medical Journal (BMJ). In any case I applied and went for interesting interviews at the Luton and Dunstable (L&D) Hospital. I first met Mr Rex Rothwell-Jackson in his office. He stood up and his head hardly moved. He was indeed a small and delightful man. Even with my lack of experience he approved of me. I then went to meet Mr Dick Fiddian, the other surgeon whose patients I would be looking after. He was completely the opposite and a very tall man. Amongst his claims to fame was that he was the regular golfing partner of Eric Morecambe, the comedian. Mr Fiddian took one look at my tie, asked me what I had done to have earned it, and then asked me when was I starting? No questions about my surgical experience at all. That morning by chance I had put on my Hawks Club tie of which I had been elected a member at Cambridge for my British Universities colours in two sports. A very lucky choice of tie as all the other members of the department of surgery had trained at Barts (St Bartholomew's Hospital) in London, but I was allowed in as a usurper. How the appointment system has now changed, and everybody has a theoretically fair assessment. Is it improved? I sometimes wonder.

The two months passed rapidly. Rex R-J, as he was unofficially known, was a superb teacher of surgery and also very sociable. Vivian (herself a Barts graduate although they did not know this when I was appointed) and I had several enjoyable evenings at his house. There were two other things that I remember about Rex. He disliked fat patients, and even more operating on them. They were therefore passed down to me. I rapidly learned that operating on obese patients is actually more difficult than on the ordinary patient. They were new to me as obese patients were then almost non-existent in Africa. The other memory was that when the SHO and I were assisting Rex during an operation he would always stand on a step so that we did not have to bend down to assist. A real gentleman with whom we kept in touch for several years until his death.

OXFORD – PLASTIC SURGERY

And then to the post as an SHO in plastic surgery at the Churchill Hospital that I had been offered whilst doing a locum as a clinical student. The hospital was

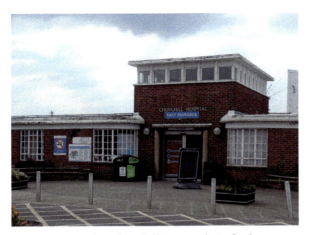

11.2 The Churchill Hospital, Oxford

situated in Headington, close to the Warneford Psychiatric Hospital and the Nuffield Orthopaedic Hospital and was two miles from the city centre. The hospital had been built in 1940 to look after orthopaedic injuries from air raids. It proved unnecessary, and was leased to the United States Army who named it after the Prime Minister, and it was formally opened by the Duchess of Kent in 1942. After the war it was handed back, and by 1974 the Churchill Hospital was somewhat of an anachronism. There was a small brick built part, but the majority of the buildings were Nissan huts left over from the second world war. (Photo 11.2) The majority of the patients were either neurology or radiotherapy patients with small surgical departments of plastic surgery, maxillofacial surgery and non-urgent general surgery. In our department there were two consultants Mr Tom Patterson and Mr John Batstone, a senior registrar and one SHO. The senior registrar was a Nigerian locum, Jim Nwozo, who had taken the place of David Evans who was spending a year working in India.

Plastic surgery had been developed as a specialty between the wars by Sir Harold Gillies. Amongst those he trained were his cousin Sir Archibald McIndoe, who became famous with his work on burned airman at East Grinstead Hospital, and Prof T Pomfret Kilner. Professor Kilner was appointed to Stoke Mandeville Hospital in 1940, and with funding from Lord Nuffield became the first professor of plastic surgery in Britain and moved to Oxford in 1944. His colleague there was Mr Eric Peet, to be followed by Mr Patterson and then Mr Batstone. I have worked out throughout my career that plastic surgeons are either scientists or artists. Mr Peet, who I did not meet, was a well recognised artist. Mr Patterson was a scientist who had published some important research. When he was operating everything would be measured. Once when we were discussing the role of private practice he said to me that he preferred his private pigs, on which he was researching, to private patients

– they argued less! Mr Batstone would look at the patient and say, as he started cutting, that that looked about right – and it almost invariably was. Another artist.

During handover from my predecessor my first job was to take his photograph to add to those of previous members of staff which were displayed on the walls. It turned out that photography was to be one of my jobs for the next six months as there was no department of photography in the Churchill Hospital and photography was, and is, of great value in plastic surgery.

I thought that I knew what to expect having done the student locum two years earlier. One of the reasons that I had taken the job was that I thought it would be a nice quiet job which would give me time to study for the Primary Fellowship examination. However, when I had done those two weeks as a locum, Mr Batstone had been on leave, and the job itself turned out to be considerably busier. It was an excellent job with a wide variety of patients, but with the exception of hand surgery and burn patients, and it gave me considerable experience of operating, both assisting and doing a minor surgery list each week. This list was for simple skin cancers and various other conditions.

The neurology unit in the hospital had an intensive care ward for patients who needed to be on a respirator. In the initial stages this was done by using an endotracheal tube in the airway. If respiration was needed for more than about ten days, then a tracheostomy in the neck was needed. One of the unusual jobs of our unit was to do these trachys, as they are known. I assisted at two of these and was then told that the next one was mine. This sounded excellent until I found that the next patient needing one was about 20 stone. The patient after that had had two previous trachys for the same recurrent problem, and the third was at last a normal trachy. Having managed the two really difficult ones with somebody looking over my shoulder, the operation never worried me in the future, and during my whole career I did more than one hundred of them.

On one occasion we had to visit a patient in Reading. Mr Batstone had had an alcoholic dinner the night before. With no warning he handed me the keys of his new, large and very expensive Mercedes. The first car of that class that I had driven.

A marvellous six months, and as I discuss later, with the input of Mr Patterson, it was the defining time of my career. With his encouragement I decided to be a plastic surgeon.

The consultants were both very sociable and Vivian and I were invited to the consultant's houses for parties and dinners. Mr Patterson was married to an artist, and their house, a beautiful Georgian house, was interestingly decorated, but definitely not in my taste! Mr Batstone had had an interesting life. After qualifying and registering he signed on as a ship's doctor and travelled around the world for some years until he met a very rich and very lovely lady. They married, and he then started training, very successfully, in plastic surgery. When he was appointed in Oxford they bought a magnificent house in Kidlington on the banks of the Thames. Tragically he developed very severe Parkinson's disease and had to stop operating and retired many years before normal retirement age. After his death their house was purchased by Sir Richard Branson of Virgin fame.

When we had arrived my wife and I had a flat in the doctor's quarters. Vivian had taken a job in a General Practice in the south of Oxford in Kennington. My post was resident on call, but it was agreed that if a home was nearby then I could be on call from there. We therefore purchased a small modern terraced house in Headington to which we moved with our six month old daughter. By buying from newspaper adverts and auctions we furnished it for £40.

I finished my six-month appointment in plastic surgery in Oxford and had two and a half months to wait for the start of the Birmingham Accident Hospital post. Needless to say I found another locum and during those eight weeks I did a locum registrar post in general surgery in Cheltenham.

CHELTENHAM

The General Hospital in Cheltenham was an elegant late Georgian building built in 1818. In the department of surgery there were three consultants, Messrs Boreham, Fairgrieve and Haynes in order of age and seniority. There were two registrars and three housemen. For a reason that I did not discover I was attached to Mr Boreham and Mr Fairgrieve and the other registrar to Mr Haynes. My two consultants gave me a wide range of surgery both to assist and to do. This included doing a clinic and an operating list each week at Telford Hospital. There my anaesthetist and my assistant were both GPs working sessions in the hospital. Before I went for the first time the strong advice from Mr Boreham was to give the GP assistant a retractor to hold, make sure that he did not move, and thank him profusely at the end of each operation.

"Do not let them operate!"

He also told me that when I was checking a patient preoperatively I must assure myself that nothing had changed and that the operation was needed. On one occasion there was a young lad of about five for a circumcision. He had had several problems in the past, but in the nine months that he had been on the waiting list these had settled. Much to the relief of the lad and his mother I cancelled the operation. Mr Boreham was not amused, but when I pointed out to him that it had been because of his instruction, he did agree.

Mr Fairgrieve was an excellent surgeon and was more relaxed. He was an interesting man and had been a previous British 880 yard Olympic runner. This had obviously caused him major problems and he had had both hips replaced before he was fifty, at a time when hip replacement was relatively uncommon.

One morning I had a call from the surgical ward letting me know that the other registrar had been admitted overnight with appendicitis. He had phoned Mr Haynes to tell him that there was a case of appendicitis which needed surgery. The reply had been,

"A private patient?"

"No – it's me."

"Well – can't you wait until morning?"

"No." was the reply.

The appendix was removed and he then post-operatively went into retention of his urinary flow. I had the unique situation of having to catheterise my colleague – luckily successfully. It also meant that until they found another locum two weeks later I was looking after all three consultants and all of their patients.

As an aside the casualty consultant at Cheltenham was an old boy from my old school, Bancroft's, called Dr Colin Flowers – but commonly known as Dr Cauliflower.

A pleasant and useful interlude with some good experience of surgery, and also living in an excellent old flat with my wife and baby daughter visiting when she was off duty.

TRELISKE HOSPITAL. TRURO

There was still a two week period before starting in Birmingham. Not to be wasted. I therefore applied for a two week locum SHO post in the accident department in Truro which had been advertised in the BMJ.

It was a very long and lonely drive from Oxford to Truro leaving behind a wife who was still working as a GP and a young daughter. The accident department was in the old Treliske Hospital which overlooked the town, and I was given a pleasant room. The department was headed by an ex-military consultant. There was a registrar and, I think, two SHOs. It was a relatively quiet job of which I have two memories. One of the duties of the on call SHO was to lead the resuscitation team. A call came from a small hospital in the centre of the town of which I knew nothing. The charge nurse said that he would show me the way, and we set off at a very high speed in my fast car. It was after all a cardiac arrest. We arrived at what was a geriatric hospital to find the patient was already in *rigor mortis,* which meant that she has been dead for at least two hours, and probably four to six. We were unimpressed by the nursing care. The charge nurse admitted afterwards that he had taken some time to recover from the drive down.

The second patient that I remember was a recently appointed consultant physician from the Royal Cornwall Hospital which had opened in 1968. He had been working in his newly bought house and had a serious injury to his left hand from a circular saw. On the staff at Truro was a very well known orthopaedic hand surgeon, Mr Robert Robins. This would have been an ideal patient for his care, but he was on leave at the time. The ex-Army accident and emergency consultant took on the case, and it was obvious to me even at that early stage of my career that he was not a hand surgeon. With my limited knowledge I could have saved two fingers that disappeared into the bin – the comment from the operating consultant was that it was a good job that he was a physician and did not need them.

The area was delightful, the natural history excellent including the birds and hundreds of adders near the coast, and I had time to drive around during my time off.

Several years later when I was a senior registrar in Leeds Mr Robins asked me to do his locum whilst he was on leave. I pointed out to him that there were a large number of orthopaedic operations that I would not be able to do. He replied that all that was needed was a hand surgeon, as none of his other colleagues were expert at the subject. I could not arrange the time off and had to turn the offer down. So regrettably I do not have on my CV, 'Locum Consultant Orthopaedic Surgeon'.

TAUNTON EAST REACH HOSPITAL

When we were working in Reading we were living in hospital accommodation and decided to buy a house of our own. We looked at properties in Norfolk, Suffolk, Dorset and Somerset and after discussions about cost and travel times we decided on Stogursey in Somerset. It was a thatched cottage, probably Elizabethan, in the centre of a row of five cottages, and definitely not in good condition. To help to pay for this I started working odd nights in the casualty department in Taunton and on some of the weekends that we were down there during the next five years.

The department was in the very elegant, but totally outdated, East Reach Hospital. The consultant in charge was Mr Cutting, and what could be a more appropriate name for a surgeon. I remember that he had been a missionary doctor in Africa and had not been able to find a formal general surgical consultancy in England on his return. The very large charge nurse in the casualty was ex military, and no patient, even when drunk, argued with him. He had a marvellous arrangement with the police. When a drunk who had been brought in had been cleared by the doctor as having no medical or surgical problem, he would carry them to the door and drop them. Before hitting the ground two policemen caught him and carted him off to the cells to sober up. Alcohol, and particularly local cider, scrumpy, was a major problem in the area. In the 1970s if 999 was dialled, the ambulance had to go to collect the patient. There was one well known alcoholic that used this regularly as a method to get a lift home. The regular ambulance drivers knew this well, but unfortunately on one occasion a new crew went out to his call. He stepped out in front of this fast ambulance and was killed.

My other memory of the hospital was a tunnel between the doctor's on-call bedroom and the department. This was always filled with cockroaches and the competition between the casualty officers was to kill as many as possible when walking through the tunnel. Eight or ten was the normal.

The hospital was replaced with a badly needed new hospital, and closed in the late 1970s, soon after my time there.

BIRMINGHAM ACCIDENT HOSPITAL (BAH OR THE ACCY)

About four months into my plastic surgery senior house officer post at the

Churchill Hospital in Oxford, during a lull in an operating session, Mr Tom Patterson the senior consultant, had asked me what I was thinking of doing in my future career. I said that my ideal was to be an accident surgeon. He pointed out that the career really did not exist in the UK, with the one exception of the Birmingham Accident Hospital.

I therefore thought about this for the next week or two, and during this time was becoming more and more interested in the variety of plastic surgery. Following another discussion with Mr Patterson I said I had decided that I would like to do plastic surgery. He obviously thought about this for a few days and then suggested I should go to the Royal College of Surgeons in London to meet Mr Dawson, who at that time was the President of the British Association of Plastic Surgeons, and very involved in the selection and training of junior doctors wanting to do plastic surgery. I therefore went to London and had a very dispiriting interview with Mr Dawson, who immediately said that he thought that I was too old to start training as a plastic surgeon.

I returned to Oxford and told Mr Patterson the result of my interview. Nothing much was said at the time, but about a week later he said that he had arranged for me to go to Birmingham to meet Mr Jackson. Mr Douglas Jackson was the senior burn consultant at the Birmingham Accident Hospital and world famous in the specialty. I therefore went to Birmingham and had a long and very interesting discussion with Mr Jackson. At Oxford we had looked after minor burns in the plastic surgery unit, as the main burn centre covering Oxford was at Stoke Mandeville Hospital near Aylesbury. I therefore had had little experience with burn treatment, and the time that I spent in Birmingham was an eye-opener. Mr Jackson took me through the field of burn treatment both nationally and particularly in Birmingham. We did a ward round to see all the patients and then had a long discussion about research. At this stage in my medical career I had published no medical research papers, and therefore the discussion was mainly about my engineering research, both with my three years in Cambridge and followed by my three years of lecturing at the University of Surrey. He obviously must have considered that I had a suitable research background because at the end of our discussion several hours later, he told me that there was a registrar job being appointed to the burn unit at Birmingham and the interviews were in three weeks. Would I please apply.

This opened a possible and completely new door for me. I discussed it with Mr Patterson when I got back to Oxford. His immediate comment was that it was a superbly useful and very lucky opportunity. I therefore applied for the job, for which I was in fact considerably underqualified as I had yet to take the Fellowship examination of the Royal College of Surgeons. Up to this point all of my posts, my house surgery post, my house physician post and my senior house officer posts at Oxford, both in the accident surgery department and in plastic surgery, had been offered to me without any of them going to an interview panel. However the requirement of the National Health Service then was that all registrar and more senior posts must be formally interviewed. This therefore was my first formal interview during my medical career. It was an interview which was certainly unlike any other interview that was to follow. Every time I could not answer a question, Mr Jackson answered it for me. Surprise, surprise I was appointed to start in June 1975.

I discovered later that Mr Patterson and Mr Jackson had been at school together and had remained in touch.

We arranged to move to Birmingham in June 1975.

As Mr Patterson had previously told me the Accident Hospital in Birmingham was indeed unique in Great Britain. After the Second World War Mr Gissane, who had been a surgeon in the British Army, wished to set up such a hospital. It meant of course that any major injury would be taken straight to that hospital, bypassing other hospitals on the way. Apparently the ambulance drivers in London had refused to agree to this, and therefore Mr Gissane set up the hospital in Birmingham with the agreement of the other hospitals in the town and also of the ambulance drivers. The medical school was founded in what had been the Queen's Hospital built in 1841 (Photo 11.3). It was situated just to the north of the Birmingham ring road, and some half mile from the city centre. In the 1970s it had 300 beds, and these were allocated to three trauma

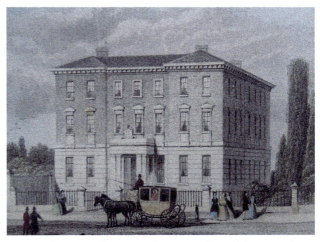

11.3 The Queen's Hospital, Birmingham. This was the original medical school and later became the famous Birmingham Accident Hospital which was the only specialised accident centre in the United Kingdom.

teams. In addition to the three teams there was a 30 bed burn unit. There were two consultants in the burn unit, Mr Douglas Jackson and Mr Jack Cason. The junior staff consisted of two registrars, and two recently qualified house surgeons. Mr Jackson had been a surgeon in the British Army.

The burn unit was the largest burn unit in Europe at that time, and already had an excellent reputation throughout the United Kingdom, Europe and the World. As well as the two surgeons, there was a famous microbiologist, Dr Edwin Lowbury whose work on the pseudomonas bacteria – at that stage the primary killer by sepsis of major burn patients – was of international importance. Amazingly he had also won the prize for being the best poet in England that year. In the pathology department was Dr Simon Sevitt, a well recognised trauma pathologist, who on first acquaintance was a somewhat difficult person, but who later became a good colleague and friend.

The burn unit was very different to virtually any other unit in the world at that time. It had been designed and created by Mr Jackson, with help in particular from Dr Lowbury, with the aim of reducing sepsis between patients, but still maintaining human connections. This was very different to the unit at the well known East Grinstead Hospital where I was to work later. At East Grinstead the patients with more major burns were completely isolated from everybody except doctors and nurses. There was no contact between patients or with their visitors, and this also applied to children. The parents were allowed to look through a window but with no physical connection. In Birmingham there were rooms for the severely injured patients in which only one patient was present. As the patient progressed they went into a room sharing with either one other patient. or as they became even better, or were more minor burns, with three other patients. There is always the problem of sepsis spreading from one patient to the other, but this connection between the two or four patients meant that they at least had a human connection and could talk to their room colleague at any time. They were not allowed into the rooms of any other patient, but they could walk along the corridor and talk through the doorway to other patients with virtually no chance of infection spreading. Other new ideas that were incorporated were that the severely injured patient rooms and the operating theatres were kept at a different air pressure so that again infection did not spread out of these rooms which were at a slightly lower atmospheric pressure. At East Grinstead there had been an interesting policy of doing the dressings in saline baths. This idea was built on a misconception which had arisen because the pilots in the Royal Air Force who had been burned and had then parachuted or come down into the sea had done better than other patients in the military. It had been assumed this was due to the salt water immersion, but was in fact due to the fact that the standard dressing for burns in the field was tannic acid. This was a very good dressing to keep infection out, but when applied, actually did more damage to the burn wound. In Birmingham the saline bath dressings had been started, but when Jackson realised that it was not of any help they had been stopped. The saline dressing bath however had been kept as a historical monument. When assisting the United States Air Force during the First Gulf War it reappeared. (see my book *Plastic Surgery in Wars, Disasters and Civilian Life*).

It turned out however that the really major change that Mr Jackson had made was in carrying out early surgery on the burn patient. When a person is severely burned, the bacteria on the surface of the skin are destroyed and the burned skin is sterile. By operating early it was possible to excise the dead skin before it became infected, and this reduced the real risk of an infection spreading into the bloodstream and killing the patient. This idea of early surgery had originally been developed by Dr Janzekovic in Czechoslovakia. She had used it on patients whose skin was only partially burned through. The dead layer of skin was excised with a graft knife and very thin split skin grafts taken from somewhere else on the patient's body were then applied and fixed in place. This work had been presented at an international conference at which Mr Jackson was present. Clearly he was suitably impressed with the results and introduced it into Britain. He then took it further in that deeper and full thickness burns were also treated with early surgery with a very considerable reduction in infection, in sepsis and in death. It was also a less painful process for the patient in that multiple dressings were markedly reduced, and the hospital stay was also much reduced. There was also less need for later corrective surgery which had previously occurred weeks, months and sometimes years after the original injury.

The burn unit had been accepted by the National Health Service as a Medical Research Council centre for research. As well therefore as the treatment of patients, research in the wards and in the attached laboratory was being carried out by Dr Bull and his team which included Drs Lawrence, Carney and Ricketts. All the team including the doctors on the wards were involved in this research which was of major international significance.

At the same interview at which I was appointed, a delightful Sudanese surgeon, Mr Hag Moussa was also appointed, and we started our appointments together.

Mr Jackson was one of the most incredible people I have been lucky enough to have met, and with even greater luck to have worked for during my life. He was not only a good surgeon, he was a brilliant innovator of new methods of diagnosing and treating the severely injured patient. As well as his surgical work, he was also a devout Christian, and was heard broadcasting regularly on the religious section of the Today radio programme. I never discovered why at quite short notice and certainly before the necessary retirement for age, he decided to retire. He was not obviously ill at that time, and I had the privilege of visiting him in his retirement in the home to which he and his wife had moved in Dorset on the south coast of England. During his life he received multiple honours in the field of surgery throughout the world. After his death, in a discussion with Dr David Herndon, the leading American burn surgeon, David said that he was astounded that he had not been recognised by a knighthood or indeed by any national honour during his life. I had the privilege of writing his obituary for the journal 'Burns' in 2004.

Mr Jack Cason was very different. He was a very capable and very fast surgeon, an extremely hard-working graduate from Leeds University who maintained a very strong Yorkshire accent throughout his life. He was academically not in the same league as Mr Jackson. He was an inveterate and very heavy smoker who eventually died from his smoking whilst still in post. His enthusiasm and rapidity of operating were well known among us, but less well-known amongst more junior anaesthetists. If the patient was brought into the operating theatre Mr Cason would immediately start operating, taking the skin grafts, at which he was an absolute and superb expert. Unfortunately the patient might not always be quite asleep or stable. Very rapidly the anaesthetists learned that the patient did not go into the theatre until they were totally sure that the anaesthetic was complete. Each year that I was in Birmingham there was a workshop for new mothers, and for those in the last stages of pregnancy. Mr Cason would give a talk with photographs about burns, how to avoid them, and what to do in the case of a burn occurring. He would then come back into the Department either smiling and rubbing his hands, saying they had to carry two or three out when they had fainted, or would come back looking miserable when nobody had had to be carried out. He did have some problems with the science of the burn injury. On occasions I remember explaining to him that a patient who had lost blood would not immediately have a low haemoglobin unless intravenous fluid had been given to him. He never could understand this although I explained it to him on several occasions, obviously not very well. His hobby was as an amateur shortwave radio enthusiast. After Mr Jackson's retirement, Mr Cason wrote a textbook on surgery which was a summary of the work and the methods that had been developed in the Birmingham Accident Hospital. He died while still in post.

As I said earlier the major trauma of the hospital was divided between three teams. Team 1 led by Mr Porter, Team 2 led by Messrs Evans and Smith and Team 3 led by Mr Peter London. After I had been in the burn unit for about one year, it was suggested that when the registrar of Team 2 was on leave that I would cover his work as well as my normal burn unit work. This was an incredible chance to receive experience and teaching in the management of trauma. The three teams were very different. Team 1 followed traditional methods of trauma management. In Team 2 both the surgeons, Mr Smith and Mr Evans were somewhat older and had a method of working by observation and by surgery only when it was obviously necessary. Team 3 was the famous team led by Mr London, who had been a very successful army surgeon, and who was a believer in very early aggressive treatment.

There were stories about all the teams. My favourite one for Team 2, who at the time had an excellent Indian registrar, was that on the ward round the day after the night on call, Mr Evans looking at a new patient asked the registrar what had happened to the patient and what had he done. The registrar said that the patient had actually cut his arm off in the middle of the night and he had put it back on joining up the bone, the vessels, the nerves and the muscles. Neither Mr Smith or Mr Evans had been informed about the patient. The immediate comment was,

"Well done, carry on."

There were multiple stories about Team 3 and my favourite one was that on regular occasions we would have soldiers from the Special Air Service (SAS) coming for training in first aid. This was obviously through Mr London's connections with the Army. We knew who the various soldiers were, but clearly the patients and the staff in the hospital did not. At one stage there was a drunken riot going on in the waiting room on a busy Saturday night. One of the SAS soldiers came to Mr London, who was operating at the time and said,

"Permission to hit one of your patients, Sir." Without looking up, permission was granted. End of riot. I do believe that that would no longer be acceptable, but it certainly worked.

I had thought the trauma consultants of Teams 1 and 3 did not really know of my existence despite two years working in the hospital. However later when

I was a registrar in Newcastle, which was my next formal appointment, Mr Jackson announced his early retirement. I was approached and asked to apply for his post. At that stage I had been qualified for only six years, and it was only two years after passing the Fellowship examination of the Royal College of Surgeons. I was interviewed, and it turned out that my main backer was Mr London, who as I said I had thought did not know me at all. It was suggested that I would be appointed, providing that the President of the Royal College would accept my appointment with my very limited experience. He didn't, and therefore I continued as a registrar in Newcastle. I was not particularly upset at the time, as my work in Newcastle was involving me in the treatment of hand injuries, and of other plastic surgery patients of whom I had had very little experience. I was in fact becoming more and more interested in both hand surgery and other forms of plastic surgery. The disadvantages of the burn unit job in Birmingham was that the work was much more limited, and it would have meant having to live in Birmingham! It would though have had the great advantage of working with the Medical Research Council unit, but this only continued to exist for about one further year in Birmingham before it was scrapped.

EXAMINATIONS

Whilst I was at the Accident Hospital I first passed the American Examination Certificate for Foreign Medical Graduates (ECFMG) examination which gave me the right to work in the States, and then passed the final Fellowship examination of the College of Surgeons. There had been excellent teaching for this at the Dudley Road Hospital by Professor Bevan, the Vice President of the College of Surgeons, and also at East Birmingham Hospital, and then a final revision course in Birmingham where I met for the first time Professor Harold Ellis. He was a brilliant teacher with a vicious sense of humour, and very unforgiving in the mock examination that ended the course. I later discovered that he was also a brilliant actor, and his viciousness was put on for the very valuable reason of giving us experience. It was said, on good statistical evidence, that the pass rate for the mock Birmingham exam was lower than that for the actual examination – and that was only 30%. I remember only one person who passed the Birmingham exam and failed the London one, but at least he passed the Edinburgh finals.

The first part of the Fellowship examination was a written paper with short answers required. Again the MCQ had not come into use by the College of

Surgeons. This was followed by a clinical examination on patients and with vivas. Much of this final clinical examination in London is still fixed in my memory forty six years later. The exam started by having to diagnose three pathology slides viewed down the microscope, and one of these was bladder bilharzia, a tropical parasite. A little unfair on the normal English doctor, but up my street as it was a common disease in Africa. There were then three vivas, a long clinical case and several short cases. There is no doubt an element of luck in exams, and it was even more so then than when I was an examiner for the same exam twenty years later. The first question that I was asked in the general surgery viva was, "How do you manage a major burn?" I started by explaining about airway problems, and that a burn completely around the chest could prevent breathing, and would need to be surgically split. The examiner looked a little non-plussed and said,

"Have you ever seen that done?" I replied,

"I did it last week."

"Where are you working," was his response, and when I replied on the burn unit at the Birmingham Accident Hospital, he said,

"I had better change the subject," and we went on to discuss haemorrhoids.

The second viva was on operative surgery and a thyroid excision was the topic. I was again lucky as I had assisted Mr Everett in several when I was working in Cambridge.

The third viva was on surgical pathology, and the examiner was Professor Herman Taylor. One of his sons was a sailing friend of mine, and I had visited the Hermon-Taylor country house in Chichester harbour. An examiner may not examine anyone that they know, but he did not instantly recognise me. We had a discussion about the chemistry of gallstones, which to a chemical engineer was right up my street.

I was worried when I saw my examiners for the long case, one was Professor Roy Calne, whom I knew from Cambridge. He immediately said that he could not examine me and introduced me to Professor Norman Browse, the President of the College. I gave a great internal sigh of relief as Roy was known to be a hard examiner. It was a little early to relax, as Professor Browse turned out to be worse. My patient was a lovely lady with cancer of the oesophagus. This had been dilated with little success. When I presented the case to Prof Browse, he asked me what I thought was the diagnosis.

"Cancer of the oesophagus, Sir."

His reply was.

"Good heavens – you wouldn't treat cancer of the oesophagus by dilatation, would you? So what do you think is the diagnosis?"

"Cancer of the oesophagus, Sir."

"Quite right my boy – misdiagnosed in the provinces."

The examiner for the final short cases I had also met briefly when I had lectured to him in Warwick about burn care. This was at the time that the BAH unit was closed for infection with typhoid and the registrars were sent around our area to give basic information to accident department staff.

After the end of the exam we all stood around in the magnificent entrance hall of the College whilst our fate was discussed. The college porter then came out with the list and called out the numbers of the successful candidates. My number was called out and I then went up to the porter who checked our names. Mr Roberts was formally used for the first time. I then went in to meet the examiners, and after signing the cheque for my membership fee, was given a glass of sherry. (Please note the order). My first examiner thanked me for my lecture on burn care which he said was very interesting. Professor Hermon-Taylor said that he thought we might have met somewhere, and I told him about a party in his house in Bosham, and the Warwick examiner also vaguely recalled having met me. Roy Calne and John Withycombe also congratulated me, and I thanked them for their teaching.

I discovered later that in the 1970s I was one of only 2½% of the candidates who passed both parts of the Fellowship first time.

When I returned to Birmingham to be congratulated by everyone Mr Jackson suggested that I deserved a holiday. After some discussion he agreed that I could use the holiday due to me and take some unpaid leave. I applied to go as medical officer on an expedition to Arctic Lapland with the British Schools Exploring Society for six weeks that summer. Whilst awaiting that decision I had to arrange the next stage of my career. To do plastic surgery I would have to have done two years as a registrar in a general surgery post fellowship, and I therefore needed a general surgery post.

SELLY OAK HOSPITAL

There was a post about to be advertised at Selly Oak Hospital in Birmingham and with support from the staff at the BAH and the other surgeons who had taught me, I applied, was interviewed and appointed. On my return from the Arctic I started at Selly Oak Hospital.

The hospital was in Selly Oak, which is a part of Birmingham three and a half miles south west of the city centre. It was originally built in 1834 as the King's Norton Union Workhouse and developed until 1948 when, on the inauguration of the NHS, it changed its name and joined the NHS. Whilst I was there a new ward block was built. Because of the stupidity of health service funding at the time there were separate budgets for construction and for running costs. The block therefore remained empty and unused for three years (Photo 11.4). A similar case was presented in the television comedy programme 'Yes Minister'. Perhaps because of this case the policy changed to a single budget soon afterwards. In 2001 Selly Oak Hospital had attached to it the Royal Centre for Defence Medicine where injured, mainly army, military personnel were admitted and treated. The hospital closed in 2011 and both the hospital and the Centre were transferred to the new expanded Queen Elizabeth Hospital. The old hospital was demolished a few years later.

In 1976 the hospital was a classical district general hospital with no specialties although it did do some teaching of medical students from the University of Birmingham. There were four general surgeons, two senior registrars, two registrars and four SHOs and house officers. I was working for

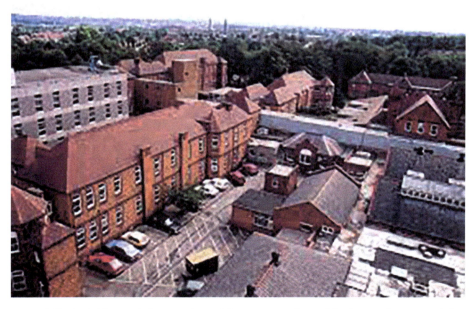

11.4 Selly Oak Hospital, Birmingham. The unopened new block is in the upper left. The hospital later had the military surgical centre aattached. The hospital has now closed and been demolished.

Mr Norman Winstone, and also looking after the patients of Mr Kaufman on on-call nights.

Mr Winstone was an interesting man. He had been a senior registrar in anaesthetics in London, and as he once explained to me he became fed up with surgeons telling him what he had to do, and therefore changed specialty. He assessed my skills in the first few days and afterwards left almost everything to me but was always willing to discuss emergency cases in the middle of the night on the telephone, and to come in when needed. On my first night on call there was a young man who had had a motor cycle accident and on examination had clearly ruptured his spleen. He needed an urgent operation to remove this to stop the bleeding to save his life. I had assisted at two of these operations previously but had never done it myself. I phoned Mr Winstone. He said get started and he would come in straight away. When he arrived, the operation was going well, and he just watched and gave me advice rather than taking over which would have been much more normal.

The work was very general surgery, but interestingly his speciality, and on which his private practice was based, was varicose vein treatment. This was ideal for me as vein surgery is not the most interesting, and nearly everything else was passed to me.

There were two other patients that had come in late at night. The first had a classical acute abdomen, and when I opened it up expecting a bleeding vessel or a leak in the gut, instead there was something inside that was completely new to me. Mr Winstone appeared, took one look, and said,

"Oh, that is abdominal TB." To which my reply was,

"And what do you do with abdominal TB?" The treatment at the time which was needed to keep him alive was explained to me. I did that, and then referred him afterwards to the physicians for treatment of the TB by drugs.

Another patient with an acute abdomen came in. He said that his tummy was a bit painful, and we held off operating. A few hours later he was much less well, and he agreed that it was a little worse. I therefore operated and found that he had clotted a major abdominal artery. I removed the dead part of his gut and put him onto anticoagulant drugs. It was a very interesting lesson. We had not realised that his origin was from the Khyber Pass area of North West Pakistan, and traditionally people from there do not show pain – even when as severe as this must have been. This is not the case in most Indian people to whom we were used, and he nearly killed himself by being so brave. The final tragedy of that patient is that some months later his GP stopped his blood thinning drugs which he needed for the rest of his life. He clotted off two more major arteries and was unsavable by the time he was readmitted.

I began to operate on both of the surgeon's patients who had gastric ulcers. In 1976 a relatively new operation had been developed to improve the situation by cutting parts of the vagus nerve which supplies the stomach instead of the whole nerve. This gave considerably fewer unwanted side effects. It was a delicate operation taking at least an hour, and ideal for a potential plastic surgeon. It was also an operation that neither of the consultants enjoyed doing and their patients all became mine. The operation was superseded by medical treatments, starting with the first H2 blockers in 1976, and rapidly improving over succeeding years. The operation no longer really exists for ulcers, but interestingly may be returning for the treatment of morbid obesity.

On another occasion I was assisting Mr Winstone with the removal of an enormous prostate gland. He had opened the lower abdomen and then passed the knife to me with the comment that the left side was easier from where I was standing. Having opened my side, I was going to pass the knife back to him. He then said that having done my side so well I may as well continue. Which I successfully did. The prostate was the size of a tennis ball and the largest that I had, or have since, seen.

I was walking through the casualty department one time and noticed a patient being pushed into the X-ray department looking very unwell. I must have been suspicious and looking at his record chart saw a rapidly falling blood pressure and a rising pulse rate. I immediately reversed the stretcher back into casualty and put up an intravenous drip which he desperately needed. Sister, who had known something was wrong when she stopped me, thanked me profusely. I then gave the young casualty officer a rapid tutorial. The casualty department in Selly Oak was of a low standard with no senior person taking an interest. This was because two miles away was the renowned Accident Hospital from which I had just come, and the theory was that all major injuries went directly there. This did mean that the casualty officers in the other Birmingham hospitals had little experience of serious problems.

Sister told me a few days later, that after my efforts almost every patient, even if it was only a common cold being treated, had an intravenous drip put in!

The final patient that I remember from there very nearly was a final patient. He was a fifteen year old lad who had been hit on the side of his head by a cricket ball. He was actually a patient of Mr Kaufmann. He asked me to see him, and on examination the lad was clearly having a major bleed within his skull which needed a very urgent operation. Because he was also a family friend of Mr Kaufmann I was asked to start the operation whilst he organised a neurosurgeon to come in urgently. In 1976 the CT scanner was just coming in nationally, and had certainly not come to Selly Oak. I started the operation and was doing the first of the burr-holes when the neurosurgeon arrived and took over. The patient survived and with no permanent loss of brain function.

As this job was coming to an end, I was looking for a registrar post in plastic surgery and was hoping that my general surgical experience would be sufficient. No jobs were advertised, and I therefore spent four months doing locum posts increasing my experience, and also hoping that one of them would lead to a permanent post. Mr Winstone knowing my needs, organised through his London connections, a two week locum for me as Senior Registrar in General Surgery at St Helier Hospital.

I remained in touch with Mr Winstone for many years. He had been a county tennis player and also a county chess champion. When I last visited him in the 1980s, he was tragically suffering from severe Alzheimer's Disease.

ST HELIER HOSPITAL, LONDON

I arrived at St Helier Hospital in Carshalton in October 1977. When seen it is immediately an unusual hospital as it was built facing the wrong way. The back faces the main road and the front a housing estate. The locum job that I was to do for the two weeks was, even in 1977, also unusual at the senior registrar level in that it was a one in one on call.

I met for the first time the two general surgical consultants,

One was very much the senior, and his greeting was,

"What can you do; boy?" Somewhat unusual in that I was nearly forty years old at the time with greying hair. I explained that I was happy with any general surgical emergency except a leaking aortic aneurysm, of which I had had no experience.

His immediate response was,

"I am sure that you will do your best – I am not available at night." It turned out that he was not available at almost any time as I did not see him again except in one clinic for the two weeks. As he disappeared, the very much younger Mr Nash said gently to me,

"I am normally available if you need me." For which I thanked him very sincerely. I found out afterwards that in the two weeks before my locum there had been three patients with leaking aneurysms, and they had all died on the operating table.

There were two patients that I remember. The first was a lady who was thirty-eight weeks pregnant with the classical history and findings of acute appendicitis except that the pain was just below her right ribs instead of in her lower right abdomen. I discussed it with the obstetrician on call and he agreed that she needed an operation. He would be in theatre with me in case she went into labour. The normal incision for an appendix would have been useless, and I therefore took out a ripe appendix through the incision for the removal of a gall-bladder. She did not go into labour, and all went well after the operation. And that was the last appendix that I have removed.

The second patient was sent to me on Friday evening with a GP's letter stating that she had had diarrhoea five times that day and he was unhappy with her condition. When we met, I asked her if she had had any more diarrhoea. She looked at me somewhat askance and told me that she had not opened her bowels for five days, and that was the reason for her visit to her GP. Both in Oxford and in Cambridge with only one exception I had been used to excellent GPs. This was my first encounter with a London GP, and discussing it with my wife, who was London trained, and with various other people I discovered that the average level of general practice in London was way below that in many other parts of England. And Friday night was when they sent in that sort of case to get rid of them before the weekend. At least the lady was easy to sort out with medicines.

My two weeks finished with some good operative sessions with Mr Nash, and thankfully no leaking aneurysms.

WEXHAM PARK HOSPITAL, SLOUGH

I was again looking for adverts for proper registrar plastic surgery posts, and for locums whilst I waited.

Wexham Park Hospital in Slough needed a three week locum in plastic surgery, and Nottingham had adverts both for a permanent post and for a two month locum leading up to it. I applied for all three, was appointed to the two locum posts, and short listed for the permanent post, with the interviews booked to occur as I started that locum.

I started the three week locum working for Mr Magdy Saad who had been there many years, and Mr David Evans, who had recently been appointed. They were both superb surgeons and of value to my training. The other person there was an elderly Associate Specialist surgeon. He was a little old fashioned, in fact old fashioned enough to be still taking split skin grafts with an unguarded graft knife. This was a technique that had disappeared many years earlier, but I will admit he performed the technique brilliantly, and it was clearly his party piece for young trainees.

NOTTINGHAM

I started in Nottingham in November 1977. The Plastic Surgery unit was in the old hospital, and we also had beds in the Children's Hospital. The new hospital was being completed, and only a few wards were open. There were two consultants, Mr Wynne-Williams and Mr Malcolm Deane. Mr Wynne-Williams was close to retirement and was not well. He was still doing clinics, but not operating. Mr Deane was much younger, and surgically very active and excellent. He was an example of the problem of the Fellowship exam. He told me that he had taken the Primary exam twelve times, never failing the same subject on a subsequent attempt. On the thirteenth attempt he passed it, and within a few weeks had completed the Finals exam with no problems at all.

The other registrar was from Saudi Arabia, and there were two house officers. These were interesting as they were in the first cohort of graduates from the new University of Nottingham Medical School.

The specialties of the unit were cleft lip and palate surgery and head and neck cancer. There was a burn unit, but no hand surgery as one of the two famous hand surgery units then in the country was in nearby Derby. This was where the sub-specialty had started in England. In the 70s, the unit there consisted only of surgeons with an orthopaedic background.

In my first week was the interview for the definitive post. I was unsuccessful. The person appointed was Miss Fiona Bailie. I was not particularly upset as she had graduated about four years ahead of me. It was also known that past registrars in the department had had to do a second registrar post before promotion to senior registrar. Towards the end of my two month appointment they did say that they regretted not having given me the job.

After I had left and when she had started, Fiona went to her bank to arrange a loan to purchase a house – and married the bank manager.

I became involved in teaching medical students, doing a weekly clinic at Mansfield Hospital, and operating at the Children's Hospital. We had an interesting weekly meeting with the pathology department. They would show the slides of the specimens excised from a patient, and then tell us whether we had got the diagnosis correct during the initial examination. It was the registrar's job to select which patients were to be discussed, and obviously we picked those that the consultants had got wrong, or that we had got right. I never did find out whether the consultants knew what we were doing. In retrospect it was useful as a teaching aid, but regrettably I never instituted it when I was a consultant.

With my previous experience and interest, I became involved with the Burn Unit which was about one third the size of the Birmingham unit. On the ward rounds, Mr Deane would walk past the door to the unit and say,

"I am assuming all is OK in there." On only one occasion did I manage to get him inside for advice.

There were two patients that I remember. The first was a teenager with a congenital abnormality of an abnormal and large collection of blood vessels in his tongue and throat. This is known as a cavernous haemangioma. These are often small at birth and then slowly grow with age. As it grew this lad was beginning to have trouble both with his speech and with breathing when he was exercising. Mr Wynne-Williams told me to put him on my operating list. For the first time I had to tell him that I had not sufficient experience to do the operation. He was somewhat upset, and Mr Deane took on the operation with me assisting. Having seen the problems that Mr Deane had, I realised how lucky both I, and more particularly the patient, had been with my refusal.

The second patient was again in Mr Wynne-Williams clinic. A lad of about eight came in with his father. Mr Wynne-Williams took one look at the lad's magnificent bat ears and said,

"I can see why you have come to see me." At which point his father said that it was actually his appointment and not his son's.

"Sir – I have been on your waiting list for twelve years – can I please swap my son's name for mine?" It was the only time that I saw a consultant so embarrassed. The names were swapped, and I did the operation a week later.

LEEDS

As I was finishing my locum in Nottingham there were no other plastic surgery locums being advertised anywhere in the country, but I did see an advert for a locum neurosurgical registrar post in the General Infirmary in Leeds. With my previous experience and interest in neurosurgery I applied and was offered the post. Some days later Professor Myles Gibson phoned me and said that the post was now a senior registrar post, which would be mine. A few days before the phone call, a locum plastic surgery post in Newcastle had been advertised. I had applied and had been offered that post. I now had two posts and a very difficult decision to make. Should I reverse my decision and do neurosurgery with the very flattering offer that had been made, or continue with plastics?

The usual arguments entered my head. A very major problem with neurosurgery is that half your patients die from brain cancer, and of the remainder, about half, are left with a permanent disability. These are clearly problems that can be difficult to deal with psychologically. This problem is very well discussed by Henry Marsh in his book *Do No Harm*. I decided to go to Newcastle. I do still wonder if I had gone to Leeds whether I would have finished up as a neurosurgeon. Had I done so there would have been an increasing element of frustration as the great skill of making the diagnosis by examination of the patient was almost completely taken over by the CT scanner, which was just coming into use. The surgery is relatively simple.

By complete chance, many years later Prof Gibson and I became friends in the Military Surgical Society. He tried to arrange for me to follow him as President, but as I had never been a serving officer, this was thought to be somewhat inappropriate.

NEWCASTLE

I drove up to Newcastle in a howling westerly gale on New Year's day 1978. Going across the North York moors in the dark, my Land Rover was moving around so much that I stopped to check the tyres and suspension. On getting out I was nearly blown away. When I arrived in Newcastle close to midnight I did not know where the Royal Victoria Infirmary (RVI) was located and asked a policeman,

"Is the hospital around here?"

"I'm not sure," he said, "but it was when I passed it ten minutes ago." After the terrible journey my sense of humour had somewhat slipped – but I did at least smile.

When I arrived I was told where to park and where the doctor's quarters were located. I found my room, and went to sleep.

In 1978 surgical care in Newcastle was split between five main hospitals, The RVI (Photo 11.5), the General Hospital, the Fleming Children's Hospital, the Princess Mary Maternity Hospital and the Freeman Hospital, the last had only opened the previous year. Plastic surgery worked in three of them. We would only visit the Maternity Hospital to see a child with a relevant congenital abnormality, and we had no beds in the new Freeman Hospital.

The consultants at the RVI were Mr Teddy Edwards, whose particular interest was in cleft lip and palate work, Mr Hugh Brown who was the primary hand surgeon and Mr David Crockford who was a general plastic surgeon both at the RVI and at the General Hospital, and also looked after the burn patients. The junior surgical staff were a senior registrar, Mr Michael Black, myself as registrar and a house officer. At the General Hospital there was one full time consultant, Mr Alan Pigott, who did general plastic surgery and head and neck cancer surgery. A second registrar was allocated to the Genera Hospital. My

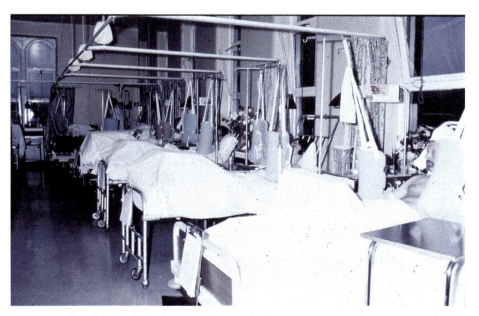

11.5 The Royal Victoria Infirmary, Newcastle. I spent two years there as part of my training.

opposite number was Carolyn Reid, whom I rarely met because the system separated us to a marked degree. Carolyn carried on in Newcastle and eventually became a consultant there specialising in the cleft work and burns. The registrars swapped jobs every six months, but at all times covered both hospitals on our nights and weekends on duty. I never discovered whether the senior registrar was officially on permanent call, but he covered both of the registrars, particularly for hand surgery problems. In general, hand injuries went to the RVI and more of the other cases and the burns to the General.

On my first morning I appeared in the RVI on Ward 5 for the ward round, and to meet the team who were based there. The ward round on any day was normally one of the three consultants, the senior registrar, the registrar, and the houseman. I had previously met the senior registrar Michael Black, at a plastic surgery meeting. The consultant and the houseman were both new to me. I was also introduced to the ward sister, Chris Allen. Although relatively young she was one of the old time, marvellous sisters. She suffered from severe rheumatoid arthritis which she valiantly ignored. I learned very rapidly that although she was quite small, the male patients on the ward did exactly as they were told, and so did we!

In every plastic surgery unit there is a mixture of acute and what are called cold cases. The latter will have been admitted from an outpatient clinic or from the waiting list. As hand surgery at the RVI was a major part of the work, acute patients formed a high percentage of the total. Two industries that have a high proportion of hand injuries are fishing and forestry, and both of these were two of the commonest industries in the north east. After surgery these patients would have their treated arm elevated in a sling, and the ward would have at least half of the patients in this condition. A major part of the post operative care often required the patient to move their fingers. In most units in the country this was controlled by the physiotherapists, but in Newcastle Sister Allen had the situation very well under control. They were told quite clearly that they were not going home until the required range of movement of the fingers had been obtained.

After the ward round I would then be allocated either to the outpatient department or to the operating theatres. Except for the three weeks at Wexham Park I had had very little experience of hand surgery. Hand surgery in the United Kingdom was, and is, split between plastic surgeons and orthopaedic surgeons. When fully trained they became members of the British Society for Surgery of the Hand. This society was 60% orthopaedic and 40% plastic. The unit in Newcastle was totally plastic with virtually no orthopaedic input at all. I therefore started my serious training as a potential hand surgeon. Mr Hugh Brown was a superb teacher in the clinic, and Michael Black a superb teacher in the operating theatre.

In the second week of my locum post the interview for the permanent post occurred. I had been very impressed with my time there and made it clear that I very much wanted the post. Very luckily they agreed that they wanted me, and I was appointed. I discovered afterwards that virtually everybody who had previously worked in the unit had been a Newcastle graduate, and I was almost the first outsider on record. I telephoned my wife and we arranged for her to come up at the weekend so that we could start looking for a house to buy, and to make enquiries about a general practice post for her.

We found an excellent house owned by a male gay couple in Jesmond which was almost next door to the Fleming Children's Hospital. It was interestingly decorated and ideal. We put in an offer that afternoon, but unfortunately that morning they had accepted a previous offer. We spent several weeks looking for another house by which time Vivian had accepted her GP post in the Durham mining villages. This put some restraint on the location of our search, and we eventually moved into a chalet bungalow, which was partly two stories, in Whickham, about one mile south west of the city centre. It had the advantage of nearly two acres of grounds which were ideal for my bird ringing and even some gardening.

At the beginning of my time there when I was on call and an acute hand injury came in, I would clerk the patient and discuss it with Michael Black. If it needed to go to theatre then for the first few weeks I would assist him, and then he would assist me for the next few weeks. After these weeks he passed my surgical skill as sufficient to be allowed to operate on my own on the acute hands. He was the perfect senior registrar as I knew that I could always call on him for advice or help. He remains a good friend.

The acute hand surgery was usually busy. The major problem was that an acute general surgical case normally took priority on theatre time, and we were nearly always at the back of the queue. This meant that we frequently did not get into theatre until nine o'clock at night or even later, and we would regularly be operating until the early hours of the morning. The other problem with the hand surgery patients was a long waiting list for the non-acute operations. I know that representations were made about this, and the unit was told that there was a theatre available, but no anaesthetist. Most hand surgery operations can be done by putting the arm to sleep with a brachial block, rather than the whole patient with a general anaesthetic. The answer was obvious – we had to learn to do brachial blocks ourselves and the registrars did so. Occasionally the block can fail partially or completely. The anaesthetist would then give a general anaesthetic, but we were not able to do this. The solution was to warn the patient that this could happen, and if it did so, we would bring them back in within a few days on a normal list. With a little experience this happened rarely, and my acquired skill with blocks has since been well used around the world.

The hand clinics with Mr Brown were interesting, and also a challenge. After I had examined the hand, he would then ask me for a diagnosis and a suggested treatment. He had taught anatomy in the earlier part of his career, and to keep up I had to really learn my hand and arm anatomy very rapidly. His diagnoses and recommended treatments were beautifully considered after alternatives had been discussed. His clinics were also great fun as he had a wealth of stories and jokes. The only slight problem was that when he was telling a joke he would start laughing before he came to its conclusion. For the first few months the jokes were new, but with new members of staff, and particularly of housemen, they were of course repeated – but still brilliantly told. After his retirement Hugh became the High Sheriff and then the Vice Lord Lieutenant for Tyneside. His wife, Ann was also a doctor and working as a GP, and her greeting on our first meeting was,

"My name is Ann." In those days of greater respect, it was an uncommon attitude.

Much of the work with Mr Teddy Edwards was with the cleft lip and palate patients. The operations for these were done in the Fleming Children's Hospital. As the registrar I would have seen the patients and their family the day before the operation, and then daily afterwards until they were discharged. If there were no cleft patients Mr Edwards would leave the list for me to do. There was an unusual anaesthetist, Dr Raymond Colback, who believed in hypnotism, even for young children. I do wonder if the reason he believed in this was that, very unusually for an anaesthetist, he was not very expert at putting a needle into small veins, and that was normally left to me. The other problem with the hypnosis was that the operating list took far longer than normal. When doing an adult list, Mr Edwards who was near retirement, on one occasion was seriously struggling, Michael Black was making slightly audible intakes of breath. Mr Edwards with his slight Welsh accent said,

"Do you think you can do it better than me?" At which point he left the theatre and Michael finished the operation far more elegantly.

On another occasion we were doing an out-patient clinic and the social worker who was there had just come back after a two month strike. She announced that she was back, and Mr Edwards comment was,

"Have you been away?" That time we were in total agreement with him as we had been puzzled why she was in the clinic at all.

A job that Mr Edwards passed to me was teaching general surgery to the dental students on a weekly basis. It was challenging, as I had to work out what were the most relevant things to teach them, particularly as their anatomic knowledge stopped at the neck, and this made life more difficult. Some weeks later I enquired whether I was paid for this. Nothing was said at the time by Mr Edwards, and afterwards Michael told me that indeed Mr Edwards was paid, but nothing had been passed on to him when he had done the job, and nothing had been passed on to me. And then to Michael's surprise two bottles of wine appeared for me.

Surprisingly there was no clinical interaction between the hospitals, but outside work it was a very sociable department, and the only consultant who did not invite us for meals or any event was Mr Edwards. We discovered why some months later when his wife was admitted having tried to commit suicide by slicing her wrists. The story which had been hidden for years then came out that she had suffered from post-natal depression for all of those years, and they had coped with this alone. We were all much more sympathetic to him afterwards and wished that we had known before as it would have made relationships much easier and could have helped them.

The third consultant who was partially at the RVI was Mr David Crockford. As well as being a general plastic surgeon he also looked after the patients on the burn unit at the General Hospital. Burned patients were a small percentage of the acute injuries at Newcastle, and this percentage was because in other units in which I had worked there were no or few hand injuries which biased the proportions of our acute work.

With my previous experience and interest, much of the burn care was handed over to me. I remember on one occasion that I was asked to come to the unit to translate for a patient. I discovered that the patient came from rural Co. Durham and the nurses said that they were having trouble as his accent was very different from Geordie. From talking to Vivian's patients on the phone I had had some experience of the dialect, but was no better than the nurses.

The sister on the unit was Margaret Robinson. She was a delightful lass whose interest outside nursing was fishing. Her family owned a shop that sold fishing equipment, and clearly had fishing rights on several rivers in Northumberland. When I was there Michael was just starting his fishing hobby, and on one round told Margaret that he had just caught his first salmon. He then asked her how she had got on in the weekend. Very gently she told him about the three large salmon that she had caught.

The General Hospital, about one mile away, had been the infirmary for the local workhouse, and had opened as a hospital in 1870. It was for many years the major hospital for the City. It became the General Hospital in 1948 when the NHS was founded, and between 2008 and 2010, all the acute services were transferred to either the Royal Victoria Infirmary or the Freeman Hospital.

In 1978 the plastic surgery unit there was run by Mr Alan Pigott. He was very much an excellent general plastic surgeon who enjoyed teaching, and for this I was very grateful. The hospital also had the neurosurgical unit for the City, and an excellent casualty department with Mr David Milne, an ex-army surgeon, in charge. On one occasion a patient was brought into the casualty who clearly had a ruptured spleen from an accident. This is a condition that needs urgent surgery. Mr Milne found that both of the operating theatres were occupied by neurosurgical cases, which were likely to be so for some time. Rather than transferring the patient to the RVI he removed the spleen from the patient in casualty whilst he was anaesthetised on a trolley, potentially saving his life.

The third hospital that we worked in was the Fleming Children's Hospital in Jesmond. This was situated a short walk from the RVI. The plastic surgery beds were shared between Newcastle and Shotley Bridge Hospital in Consett, Co. Durham. Plastic surgery at the Fleming had an interesting history. It had been started by Mr Fenton Braithwaite (1908 – 1985), who after the war, started plastic surgery in the north of England with Mr Edwards as his registrar. Mr Braithwaite was a remarkable man. He had read mathematics at Manchester and he then changed to medicine at Cambridge and St Bartholomew's Hospital in London, qualifying just before the war in 1937. He served in the RAF during the war, and then moved to East Grinstead under Sir Archibald McIndoe, becoming a plastic surgeon and doing some important research. In 1959 he was appointed to the north east to set up a service, and this included his special interest of cleft lips and palates at the Fleming. When I was there in 1978 he would often drop into the tea room to talk to me between cases, as he was clearly missing not operating. I only discovered later his special interest and knowledge in old scientific books and also antique furniture, but unfortunately they never came into the conversations as I would have been very interested to have seen them. His other interest was in Newcastle United Football Club, of which he became Life President in 1983, and to whom after his death he apparently left his large fortune.

I have already mentioned that Mr Edwards had taken over the Newcastle cleft palate work and I would on occasions assist him. Mr Bell, the senior plastic surgeon from Shotley Bridge also operated on the cleft children from there.

My interest in the Fleming deepened when I discovered that 90% of the paediatric urgent waiting list consisted of children with hypospadias, and that no one was operating on them. Hypospadias is an unusual congenital condition occurring in 1 in 80 male births in England in which the opening of the penis is not at the end but somewhere along the shaft. I discussed this with Mr Edwards who said that neither he nor his colleagues wanted to be involved, and why did I not take an interest. I discovered that Mr Crawford at Fulwood Hospital in Sheffield was the local expert. I contacted him, and was invited to Sheffield to discuss the condition, its treatment, and complications, and to see him operate and assist. This I did for a day a week for three weeks, and then started with some relatively minor cases at the Fleming. Hypospadias repair is done in a one stage operation for mild forms, and a two stage operation for the worse cases. The two stage operation cases commonly have a complication where there is a leak mid shaft, called a fistula. I did all the one stage operations on the waiting list without any problems. I then noticed that there were several boys on the urgent waiting list with fistulae from previous operations. I had discussed similar cases with Mr Crawford, for which there was no known simple operation. I therefore worked out a possible method of repair that I tried out on some cases which gave good results. The ward sister told me that there had been a large number of problems with some of Mr Bell's patients. I asked him if I could use my new operation on some of these patients, but he declined.

Close to the end of my two years Mr Bell retired and his place was taken by Mr Gus McGrouther. We had met at various conferences and had got on well, and this was the start of a long association, particularly with research.

Patients that I remember well included one of the first patients that I saw in a clinic. I asked her what was the problem, and she replied,

"I have a lump in my lisk."

Not having a clue as to where was her problem, I thought for a few moments, and then said,

"Show it to me." The lisk is a very specific Geordie word for a groin. I had come across oxters before, but lisk never. (Oxters are armpits from Yorkshire up to Scotland).

And there are always disasters that lodge in one's brain. A terrible one was an elderly lady who had received severe burns. After several skin grafting operations, she was discharged home. The ambulance taking her home crashed, and tragically she was killed.

A forester was brought in as a serious emergency. He had been using a chainsaw and hit a piece of metal in the log. This caused the saw to rebound and it split his face and head almost vertically in the midline. By the time he arrived in casualty the bleeding had been stopped, but he was still leaking cerebrospinal fluid from around the brain. When I explored the wound at operation, I found that the tissues surrounding the brain had been cut, but the brain itself was intact. I repaired the various layers, reconstructed the nose, and sutured the rest of his face and his lips. He recovered well and I saw him three months later in a clinic. He was back at work with an almost normal looking face with a good cosmetic scar. He was extremely grateful and thanked me for my efforts.

There were three other patients whose injuries were almost unbelievable, and they may be a world record as they had happened on the same day. The first came in just after lunch having cut off his thumb. Michael Black had recently returned from a year learning microvascular surgery in Melbourne, Australia, and with my very inexpert assistance was replanting it. As the operation was coming to the end four hours later, I had a call to go urgently to casualty where Mr Maitra, the casualty consultant of the RVI, showed me a second patient also without a thumb. I went back to theatre and told a weary Michael about the case that was to be the next on the list. When he was finishing that, another four hours later, back to casualty I went for the third case. This man had not quite cut his thumb off completely, but had cut both arteries and both nerves, which made the operation almost identical. Back to theatre I went and said to Michael,

"You are not going to believe this, but we have a third case." He did not, and it took me some time to convince him. Thanks to Michael's skills all three thumbs survived. How long Michael took to recover I never did discover.

In my last few months three things happened which might have affected my future career. It was suggested that I applied for a year as a Fellow in the

Microvascular Unit in Melbourne, the same post that Michael had held. I was told that these were normally reserved for people who had already been appointed as a senior registrar. One of my referees must have said nice things about me as I was offered a fellowship starting eighteen months later.

The second opportunity was to spend two months as a locum senior registrar at the renowned East Grinstead Hospital. My report on this two months follows later.

I had also applied for a senior registrar post in Ireland. I was called for an interview for the post in Dublin. I went across the sea and spent a day looking around the units before the interview. It was a tough interview which I enjoyed, and I thought that I had done well. Afterwards they said that they had been impressed, but they were going to appoint their local man, Denis Lawlor – but in typical Irish fashion, would I please take his job as a locum for two years whilst he first went to Melbourne for microvascular training, and then somewhere else for a second year. A difficult decision as the two years were all that I needed to be able to apply for consultant posts, but if unsuccessful at interviews I could be left in limbo. I decided to turn the offer down. A few weeks later I was appointed to the senior registrar position in Leeds and Bradford.

"Ee – you are going to the south then," was the farewell statement from the nurses – and they meant it. To a Geordie, Leeds is definitely in the south.

I very much enjoyed Newcastle. The plastic surgery unit, although split geographically, worked well. The house officers were the best that I came across anywhere, and the nursing was excellent. Within the RVI there were obvious divisions in some of the other units, and the professor of surgery Professor I D A Johnston was not altogether popular. It was said that at one of the Christmas medical student shows that his initials stood for 'I Decide All Jobs', and this upset him as it stuck rather permanently.

Newcastle introduced me to hand surgery, and with Hugh Brown teaching me what to do, and Michael Black teaching me how to do it, there could not have been better instructors. Encouragement and trust in my abilities in hypospadias surgery started me in the specialty which continued throughout my career. I also appreciated the attitude of the Geordies – 'Thank you for coming to work up here', which was so different to some other places in which I had worked. I will always be extremely grateful for those two years.

Certainly the weather did play a part in life there. It was said that when one ceased to comment on the howling westerly winds which blew almost daily, that one had become a local. The winter of 1978/9 is remembered not only for the snow, but also that the road cleaners/gritters were on strike. Even with my Land Rover I had to walk four miles into and back from the hospital for a few days. Patients arrived by tractor and by horse. Vivian in her practice in old mining villages in Durham with a large number of working nights, and often very bad weather was unfortunately less happy, but we survived well. I also drove Vivian out to her patients on occasions as her usual road was under a 17 foot deep snow drift.

EAST GRINSTEAD

The plastic surgery and burn unit at the Queen Victoria Hospital had become world famous during the second world war for the work of Sir Archibald McIndoe on the airman of the allied air forces who had been burned – mainly in crashes. Much of the fame was because of the innovative reconstruction, but Sir Archibald and the anaesthetist Dr John Hunter also recognised the importance of social interaction, both with the staff and between the patients, and also within the local residents. The patients founded the Guinea Pig Club amongst themselves in 1941, and even the local public house (demolished in 2009) later adopted the name. Whilst I was there the club was still functioning with an annual dinner, but in 2022 almost all the members have now died. McIndoe deserved his reputation, but also had luck on his side. The majority of his patients were young and had been very fit before their accidents, and as Lord Beaverbrook was a friend, he had excellent publicity in the national press. There are available many books about his work and the Club, and there is a commemorative museum in the village. He died in 1960 aged only 59, and just before he became the President of the Royal College of Surgeons.

My two months of July and August in 1979 at East Grinstead were an almost complete contrast to my previous plastic surgery experience. The unit was in a small specialist hospital which it shared with a maxillo-facial unit and an ophthalmic unit. There were five consultants and normally five junior trainees who were either registrars or senior registrars. Each one of these was attached to one consultant. When I joined there was a vacant post, and I was allocated to be shared between Mr John Cobbett and Mr Nick Breach. It was a lucky posting as my two consultants were excellent and had specialist interests.

Mr Cobbett had had his early plastic training from Sir Archibald, and specialised in hand surgery. He had done the first successful microsurgical toe to thumb transfer in the world in 1968. On first acquaintance he was a shy man, but became easier to talk to after the first few days. He was an excellent surgeon and teacher. One of his stories was about a piece of jewellery that one of his grateful Arab patients had given him. He was not impressed with it and was about to give it to his eight year old daughter, but luckily took it into a jeweller first. Having been told that it was worth many thousands of pounds, he sold it, and bought something else for his daughter.

Mr Nick Breach was a very different character who made me feel instantly at home. He had originally trained as a dentist and became a maxillo-facial surgeon, and then changed to medicine. His interest was in the treatment of cancer. As well as East Grinstead we also did a clinic in Brighton. I had always thought that Brighton was a civilised town but what astonished me was the number of patients who had let their skin cancers grow to an enormous extent without seeking help. At operations between us on these patients we often had to remove eyes or reconstruct eyelids. At Brighton there was an elderly dermatologist, Dr Patrick Hall-Smith who ran his clinic next to ours. He had a habit of taking a small biopsy from an obvious tumour for histology, and then sending the patient to Nick for the treatment that was obvious in the first place. I know that Nick tried to convince him that this was unnecessary, and entailed an extra operation, as well as delaying that operation, but I never did discover if he succeeded. The clinic finished with a pleasant lunch in a pub on the way back to East Grinstead. Clearly the post at East Grinstead was not what Nick wanted, and soon after I left he moved to the Royal Marsden Hospital in London and became a full time cancer reconstructive surgeon.

As I have said earlier the burn unit was unique, and had changed little over the years since Sir Archibald. If I had a phone call referring a potential patient the first thing that I had to do was check that there were sufficient nursing staff able to cope. This problem was exacerbated as each burn patient, and even those with relatively minor burns, was in an individual cubicle. This required more nursing care than had been the case at the other units in which I had worked, and had the second disadvantage that no visitors were allowed into the cubicle. This also applied to the parents of children.

There were three other plastic surgery consultants Messrs Cochrane, Bennett and Bowen, one other senior registrar, Peter Davenport, and two registrars. One was an excellent New Zealander whom I was to visit later.

I remember an eighteen year old young man in the clinic who had had a congenital hypospadias. This had been operated on unsuccessfully several times, and he was still having to sit to pass water. Using my operation I operated on him successfully. When I saw him in the clinic four weeks later, he was very grateful, but still unnecessarily sitting down to pass his water. I tried to encourage him to try standing up but as I was only at EG for a few weeks, I lost touch and do not know if I succeeded.

Also within the unit was a very interesting consultant anaesthetist, Dr Hale Enderby who had developed, and was the world expert, in hypotensive anaesthesia. At operation the blood pressure was intentionally lowered in an attempt to reduce blood loss and therefore the necessity of blood transfusion in major reconstructive surgery.

There was a strong social life with a bar to which nearly everybody dropped in on the way home at the end of the day. The barman was definitely a character. When in the RAF during the war he had been posted to East Grinstead and employed as a theatre assistant to Sir Archibald (The Boss) amongst others. One of his jobs was to sharpen the skin graft knives. The Boss would always complain that they were not sharp enough and pass them back. After about the third rejection the original, and untouched knife, was passed back and accepted as much better. When he had retired as a theatre assistant he just kept coming back to run the bar. At some stage he had married one of the hospital cleaners, and when I got to know him better, I discovered that he and his wife owned and rented out some five or six properties in the town. A rich barman indeed.

Having come from the extremely busy Newcastle Unit there was spare time in the evenings to write. In my first week there I wrote two papers summarising my work on hypospadias from Newcastle and my fistula operation. They were both accepted for publication without a word being changed.

My final memories of East Grinstead were the Guinea Pigs. At a meeting whilst I was the SHO at Oxford I had heard Geoffrey Page describe hie experience as a Guinea Pig, and that had inspired me. He wrote about this in his book *Tale of a Guinea Pig*. I also met several of them at EG, and at meetings elsewhere. One that I got to know a little was Dr Sandy Sanders. He had been badly burned in a Tiger Moth crash and reconstructed. The experience was such that after the war he became a medical student and then a GP in Shropshire, He was one of the last surviving Guinea Pigs. They were remarkable people.

And then I went back to Newcastle to discover that two senior registrar posts in Leeds and Bradford that were advertised.

LEEDS/BRADFORD

I visited both units, and with five other candidates was interviewed in Harrogate. I gratefully accepted the post when it was offered to me, and it was agreed that I could have the year away in Melbourne. David Sharpe was the other candidate appointed at the same interview. I gave my two month statuary notice, we put our house on the market, and started looking both for a house which would be convenient for both units, and also for a GP practice for Vivian.

In an unusual way the Yorkshire set up was similar to that in Newcastle. The differences were that the two units were ten miles and not one mile apart, and it was the senior registrars rather than the registrars that rotated – this time on a yearly basis. Again there were no clinical or educational contacts between the units.

In March 1980 David started in Leeds, and I went to Bradford for a year. The Bradford unit was based at St Luke's Hospital and consisted of two consultants, Mr Tom Barclay and Mr David Crockett, the rotating senior registrar, a registrar and two SHOs. Although Mr Barclay was the co-author with Ian Muir of the standard textbook on burn care, the unit took only minor burns as all the major burns went to the regional burn unit at Pinderfields General Hospital in Wakefield to be looked after by Dr John Settle. The unit also rarely took hand surgery patients unless there was major skin loss. The hand surgeon at the Bradford Royal Infirmary, the other hospital in Bradford, was Mr Bill Holms with whom we had occasional contact.

St Luke's Hospital had been built as the workhouse infirmary in 1852. It was used as a military hospital in the second world war and joined the NHS as St. Luke's Hospital in 1948. When I was there it covered mostly medical specialties and the only surgical specialties were plastic surgery and maxillo-facial surgery – both adult and paediatric. It was certainly Victorian and had been little improved. The photograph (11.6) is of a patient being wheeled from the children's ward to the operating theatre on a rainy day in the winter.

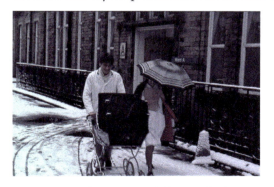

11.6 St Lukes was an old hospital. The photo shows a child being wheeled from the children's ward to the operating theatre.

The two consultants were both very different and were very interesting characters. Mr Barclay was the senior and the organiser of the unit. He either approved of one, or didn't. Grey did not exist between his black and white. When I joined the unit he had not liked my predecessor, and did not like the registrar. Very luckily, he approved of me, and this meant that my clinical and operating skills were widely used from the start. He was an excellent opinion and a good surgeon. What was most unusual for a senior surgeon was that he would either read or hear about a new technique from anywhere in the world, and then introduce it on a trial basis in Bradford. Even more interesting from our point of view and experience was that it was the senior registrars who did the operating. When I was there for my second time after my year in Australia, we were one of the first units in England to use tissue expansion, and also to use fasciocutaneous flaps. Bill Dickson was the SHO at the time, and with the encouragement of Mr Barclay, we published papers together on the uses and complications of both the techniques which are now widely used in the United Kingdom and around the world.

Mr Barclay occasionally asked me to operate on his private patients. I learned later that he would tell the patient that his senior registrar did the operation better than him, and if they were agreeable I would do it. In particular I did hypospadias repairs and block dissections of the groin and of the axilla for cancers. I was also grateful that he paid me well for my services, and even more grateful that none of them went wrong. There were two other interesting facets of Mr Barclay. He was a superb politician, and whilst I was there was elected as President of the British Association of Plastic Surgeons. He was also an avid and excellent golfer to the extent that on the Monday morning ward round we had to discover whether he had won or lost that weekend. If he had lost the ward round was very quiet. If he had won, we could chat merrily. In the summer he would play three or four holes before the ward round at 0900hrs, and a few more holes on the way home. Playing with his son, a full-time GP, who had a handicap of one, one year they were fourth in the national Father and Son British championship. The other nine pairs in the top ten were all professionals. Tom retired from the NHS at 60 with a handicap of four, and at the age of 70 still had the same handicap.

Mr David Crockett was very different. A delightful man and a good surgeon who smiled happily as the world went by. When younger he had had a series of operations for a benign brain tumour. After these, and probably caused by the surgery, he was according to his wife, much more benign. He could not always have been benign as he had a Cambridge Blue for judo! He had also worked in the Sudan for several years when there were no jobs being appointed in the United Kingdom. In Bradford, we would do operating lists together – or to be more precise he would do one case and I would do the rest while he either read his New Scientist or did medico-legal reports in the changing room, popping into the theatre every so often to see how I was doing, and offering the occasional advice. He was also helpful with research, suggesting two topics, and both pieces of work were later published.

It was a very sociable department with constant interactions with the consultants, and also with David Sharpe. Until the Bradford Fire we had never worked together but we became good friends.

In my second spell in Bradford, our SHO, Sonia Banerjee became pregnant. She gave up her post and did a successful research degree at the University of Bradford which I supervised. There were two interesting parts of this work. The research was based on rats, and one day whilst I was in the animal house talking to the senior technician, he was clearly having a heart attack in front of me. I sent him off to the cardiac unit. I heard afterwards that when he arrived, he denied all knowledge of being unwell. Luckily I had phoned through to tell them he was coming and the ECG did indeed show a new infarct. He responded well to treatment and even gave up smoking. The second interesting occasion was Sonia's graduation ceremony. Harold Wilson was the Chancellor awarding degrees, and unfortunately his address was partly excellent and partly confused. Alzheimer's disease had started and that was his last public speech.

After six months Vivian and I set off for the year in Australia. (Chapter 12). On my return I went to Leeds for six months before returning to Bradford for a complete year.

The Leeds unit was somewhat different as were the hospital arrangements in Leeds. Again there were two main hospitals, and also several smaller specialist hospitals.

Plastic surgery was based in St James's Hospital (Jimmys) to the north-east of the city. At the time Jimmys had about 1,600 beds, which was more than any other hospital in Europe. Plastic surgery also had beds, particularly for children, at the Leeds General Infirmary. Jimmys had been founded in 1848 as the Leeds Moral and Industrial Training School. It then added a workhouse in 1858, which included an infirmary. In 1925 it was renamed St James's Hospital in memory of a previous medical superintendent and a former governor. An unusual choice of name as neither was a Saint. In the First World War it was a war hospital, and then joined the NHS in 1948. A further change of name occurred in 1970 when on the expansion of the medical school it became St James's University Hospital. It was an enormous hospital, and because of this rather unfriendly. Plastic surgery shared a separate wing with the orthopaedics and the maxillo-facial surgical units and almost the only people from outside were the visiting anaesthetists. To go to the doctors' mess for lunch was not worth the effort as it was a ten minute walk each way, leaving only ten minutes to buy and eat the food.

The Leeds General Infirmary (LGI) was close to the city centre. It was founded in 1767 as a hospital for the sick and poor of the parish. It outgrew the site, and in 1868 a new magnificent building designed by Sir Gilbert Scott was built on an adjacent site. Several wings have been added since, and now in 2022 it is much larger than it was in 1980, but still smaller than Jimmys. In 1980 plastic surgery had one paediatric operating list there each week.

The unit in size and the type of cases was similar to Bradford. Major burns went to Dr John Settle in Wakefield, and the hand surgeon was Mr Robert Brown, a South African orthopaedic surgeon. There were two plastic surgery consultants, a rotating senior registrar and two SHOs.

Again the consultants were very different to each other. Very much the senior was Mr Derek Eastwood. He was a superb surgeon and a complicated character. Whatever he did, and whatever we did, was never quite right. The out-patient sister was marvellous, and used to warn the patients when they came back for their post-operation visit that Mr Eastwood would always say,

"That's not quite right – I should have done a little more."

In fact the only person who could see anything wrong at all was Mr Eastwood. In my two years there, only twice did he say well done to me – and I gather that was more than usual. The most unusual surgery that he did were sex-change operations. He had become involved in these because a psychiatrist had asked him for his help, and because the female to male operation was, and is, extremely difficult he found the challenge stimulating. Very tragically whilst I was there two patients on whom he had operated very successfully both committed suicide in the same week. He decided that he had been wasting his time and did no more sex interchange surgery. I only saw one mistake from his surgery where he had put on a bandage that was too tight after an hypospadias operation, causing some skin loss. After that I did all the hypospadias children on his waiting list. He taught the medical students, but would never lecture or present a paper at a meeting as he told me that it would make him stammer. Outside surgery his great interest was in opera, and when attending a meeting in London would go to an opera rather than attend the official conference dinner.

The second consultant was Mr Chips Browning. He had just been appointed when David and I started and one of us took the post that he had just left. I had the impression that both David and I had by chance done more surgery in our respective training than had Chips, and this initially made a slightly restrained relationship between us. This improved over the years. He took on the paediatric work at the LGI. In my second spell at Leeds a new consultant paediatric surgeon was appointed to the LGI. He was obviously interested in taking over the hypospadias patients and he and Chips compared their post-operative fistula rate. Ours was much lower than his. He then asked if he could come and learn from us before taking over the work. Chips made it very clear that we were not giving up the hypospadias kids and he would not be welcome. I remember one amazing case which appeared in the clinic. Three young boys from the same family were born with hypospadias – and the father also had the condition. All four were offered a correction. Father said that although he knew that hypospadias could reduce his fertility rate, it clearly had not done so, and he would do without a correction. The three boys we did one after the other on the same list, and all with success.

Another case that I remember was a man that had a major injury to a leg. Chips and I had done a microvascular flap to give good skin cover, and he was due to have a bone graft by an elderly orthopaedic surgeon. I was sent along to ensure that that surgeon did not damage the blood supply to our flap. I was scrubbed up and just managed to preserve our flap from his intentions, although it was a close run thing. The graft was successfully done, and I started suturing up the skin with 3/0 Prolene sutures. The orthopaedic surgeon, looking askance, asked if I thought that the suture was strong enough. I assured him that this was the type and size of the suture that we routinely used. He asked for the same and started suturing the other end of the wound. At the end he gave the area a clean, and unfortunately all his sutures fell out. At which point he left the theatre, and I finished the operation. He was clearly only familiar with silk sutures which tie more easily, but do have a slightly higher risk of infection.

One of Chip's outside interests was as medical officer to the Headingly Rugby Football Club. On Monday morning the ward round often started with one of the rugby players who had come to be assessed, and when necessary put on the operating list for the injury that he had sustained on the Saturday to be properly repaired. His other interest was fast cars.

On my return from Australia, I was looking for microvascular cases to keep my newly acquired skills in practice. I did several replanted fingers and then Mr Eastwood suggested that I could do a transplant from the scalp to the upper lip of a young man. He had had an electrical burn to his mouth as a child and was extremely embarrassed by his scarred and non-moving lip. I discussed the operation and the complications, and he asked me to go ahead. It was successful and he was well satisfied with the result.

I have said earlier that the requirement to be eligible for an NHS consultant post was two years as a senior registrar. My year in Australia did not count towards this. There was a second requirement to keep the senior registrar post renewing itself in that one had to apply for a reasonable (but undefined) number of the jobs that were advertised. All the senior registrars were well aware of these conditions. During the year after my return from Melbourne, Mr Brown phoned me from Newcastle. They were hoping to have approved a new consultant post there, and if so, would I be interested. For me it was the perfect post with a mixture of hands, burns and microvascular surgery in a very active department. I said that I would indeed be interested, and he then said that the job description had been written for me, but the only problem was that the funding had yet to be agreed. One year later the conversation was repeated – but still no funding. Mr Brown suggested that I could take a post at Shotley Bridge Hospital, and then transfer when the job was funded. I was less happy with this as it would have meant changing houses, schools and Vivian's jobs, and decided not to take up the offer. I held on for that job for another year, but was having to apply for other consultant posts elsewhere.

The succession of job applications is of interest. There was an advertisement for a post in Liverpool at the Whiston Hospital. It was certainly not a post that I wanted, and we all knew that John Stillwell, who was the senior registrar in post, wished to be appointed to the post. I therefore applied. In the train going to Liverpool, I met Mr Hugh Brown, my old boss from Newcastle, who was the external assessor. I tried to make it clear to him that I did not wish to be appointed to this post. Unfortunately the job description could almost have been written for me as it contained burns and hand surgery. In the interview I was clearly getting on well with the interview panel. In those days the appointment was made and announced on the same day at the end of the interviews with all the candidates present. Normally the discussion behind closed doors would take fifteen to twenty minutes, but on this occasion as time elapsed, and became above one and a half hours, I was becoming extremely worried that the appointment might come my way. At last, the secretary to the committee came in and announced "Mr Stillwell". It is the only interview to which I have ever been where everyone smiled at the result, John because he was being appointed consultant, and the rest of us because we weren't. Quite rightly Mr Brown never did tell me about the discussions that went on behind the scenes.

Very soon after the Liverpool interview, a job became vacant at Great Ormond Street Children's Hospital in London. Of all the places in Britain, London was the one place that I did not wish to be appointed. I therefore did not carry out what was then a necessity of a preparatory visit to the hospital to talk to the people in post and to work out what the job included. I was delighted when I was not shortlisted, but at least I had applied for another job, and that was what mattered at the time.

The next post that became vacant was at St Andrew's Hospital, Billericay in Essex. In many ways this was again an almost ideal post for me in that it involved running the very well known burn unit, but also included some head and neck surgery which was not one of my sub specialties. I went to see the job, and had an interesting and very useful tour of the hospital. It turned out, however, that part of the job was operating at Whipp's Cross Hospital in Wanstead. I visited Whipp's Cross Hospital (which I had known as my mother had died there, and where I was also treated for a broken wrist as a child when at school). The plan there was to do a clinic in the morning, operate in the afternoon, and then not go back to the hospital for another week. I enquired who looked after the patients on whom one had operated. I was told that the general surgical juniors would do this and call one if there was a problem. This I was convinced was not the best way to treat one's patients who one had just operated on, as help would by then be thirty miles away. I therefore decided not to apply for that post.

The next post that came up was at the famous East Grinstead Hospital in Sussex. We all knew that the senior registrar in post, Trevor O'Neill, desperately wanted the job. I had spent two months as a locum senior registrar at the hospital, and was not really convinced that I did want the job, although again it did have a burn unit with what were at that time some unusual and rather dated practices. At the end of the interviews, the secretary came into the waiting room where all those who had been interviewed were waiting, and announced "Mr Tanner". The look on the face of Trevor was of a person totally shattered. And I think we were also feeling very much the same as this was a very unusual outcome. Trevor later went on to become a very successful consultant in the Norwich hospitals.

And then came the advertisement for the consultant post at Stoke Mandeville Hospital, for which I successfully applied.

TWELVE

MICROSURGERY IN AUSTRALIA

This chapter and the next are summaries. This period in Australia and my subsequent career have been fully described in another volume of my memoirs: *Plastic Surgery in Wars, Disasters and Civilian Life* which is about to be published.

An operating microscope had been used in ophthalmology for many years. In the 1970s and 1980s the technique started to be used to join small blood vessels and lymph vessels by plastic surgeons. It made possible replanting limbs and even digits which had been cut or pulled off. With practice a trained microvascular surgeon could join together arteries, veins or lymph vessels with an external diameter of 0.5mm. At that time there were major developments in the understanding of the anatomy of the skin and using the microscope made possible movement of skin and other tissues around the body. This was a considerable advantage to the older method of joining pieces of skin to other parts of the same patient's body, and then transferring the part by separating it three or more weeks later from where it had originated.

Microvascular surgery training did not really exist in the early 1970s. English surgeons who included John Cobbett at East Grinstead and Bruce Bailey at Stoke Mandeville had learned the technique in the laboratory themselves. By the mid 1970s two places in the world had set up training facilities. One was in Melbourne, Australia by Bernie O'Brien and one in Louisville, Kentucky in the United States by Harold Kleinert. Michael Black had been the senior registrar in Newcastle when I was the registrar, and Chips Browning was the new consultant

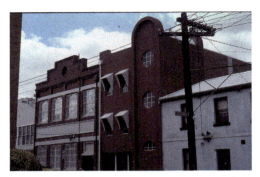

12.1 The O'Brien Microsurgery Research Centre attached to St Vincent's Hospital.

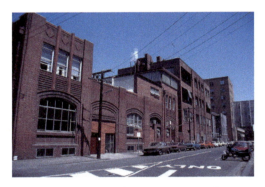

12.2 St Vincent's Private Hospital, Melbourne, Australia.

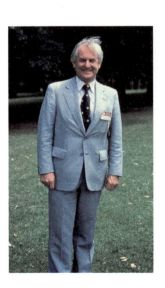

at Leeds. They were two of the four British trainees that had spent a year in Melbourne learning the technique. Although theoretically not senior enough I had applied to Melbourne and was offered a Fellowship to start eighteen months later.

And so in June 1981 my wife, two daughters and I set off to Australia taking a month to get there visiting friends in the Philippines, Malaysia, Thailand and Brunei on the way. We then had to find a house, a car, schools for our daughters and some locum work for Vivian. I started in the famous microsurgical laboratory (Photo 12.1) attached to St Vincent's Hospitals (Photo 12.2) working with Bernie O'Brien (Photo 12.3) and the other plastic surgeons in the hospital, and particularly Wayne Morrison. The work started in the lab learning the technique and then incorporating a research project, and very soon moved into assisting and then doing clinical cases. Details of some of these and the other aspects of the year are in *Plastic Surgery in Wars, Disasters and Civilian Life*.

One extremely rare case was a young fourteen year old girl who had caught her hair in the back

12.3 Mr Bernie O'Brien. My senior consultant in Australia. One of the major founders of microvascular surgery throughout the western world.

12.4 A major microvascular replant following the loss of her scalp in a farming accident.

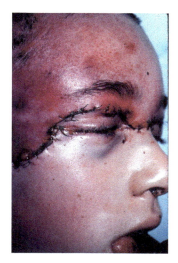

of a tractor and the whole of her scalp, forehead and one ear had been pulled off. Twenty four hours of surgery by two consultants and two fellows and it was replaced (Photo 12.4). Without the success her life would have been devastated. Because of the successful replantation two years later she became a model.

A challenging, fabulous year and a technique well worth learning which I was able to use for the remainder of my career and in several countries. We also had the opportunity to see some of Australia including Ayre's Rock (Photo 12.5).

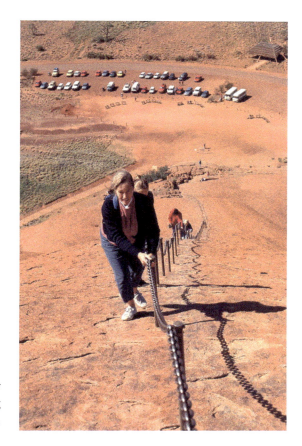

12.5 Ayre's Rock. My family climbing - or at least walking up it. This is no longer possible.

THIRTEEN

CONSULTANT AT LAST

In 1985 I was appointed as a consultant plastic and hand surgeon at Stoke Mandeville Hospital near Aylesbury, and with the added role of Director of the Oxford Region Burn Unit (Photos 13.1, 13.2 and 13.3). The thirteen years of my training that led up to this has been described in the earlier chapters. The general surgery training that I had had both in England and overseas was very useful, both to give me confidence, and also to combine that with the specialised plastic surgery that I had also learned. The plastic surgery training which matched my interests in the treatment of burns and of hand injuries were ideal for the job that had been advertised. I was even luckier to be offered time to continue with the research which complemented the quite extensive research that I had done, and with papers published.

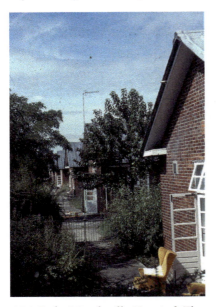

13.1 Stoke Mandeville Hospital. The wartime units with an underground air raid shelter between each ward.

The consultant appointment within the National Health Service in the United Kingdom and Ireland differs from almost any other career. For the first time one has the responsibility for the total care of any patient who is registered under you. There is of course the requirement that this care must be within both legal and professional limits laid down by the General Medical Council and by the College(s) to which one belongs. Although it seemed a long and intensive period as a junior, I was at the time the second fastest trainee through the system in plastic surgery. I was still in post as a senior registrar in Yorkshire and immediately handed in my notice. Part of my contract there was that I had to work for a three further months. During

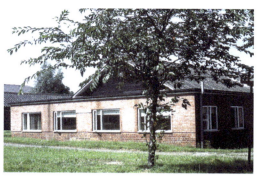

13.2 The back of the old Burn Unit. The second oldest burn unit in England opened by Sir Harold Gillies in 1956.

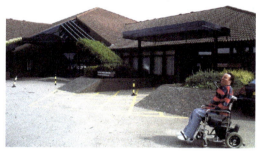

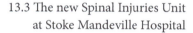

13.3 The new Spinal Injuries Unit at Stoke Mandeville Hospital

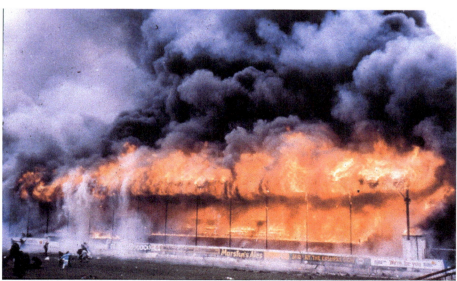

13.4 The Bradford Football Stadium fire. May 11th 1985.

this period the Bradford Football Club fire occurred on the 11th of May 1985 (Photo 13.4). A date carved into my heart and brain. This disaster altered my future career both from the actual experience, and also from the subsequent travels around the world to an incredible degree.

The Bradford Fire and my subsequent career have been fully described in the volume of my memoirs entitled: *Plastic Surgery in Wars, Disasters and Civilian Life.*

Part Three
Sport

INTRODUCTION

From the age of eighteen sport became more and more an essential part of my life and of my success, and this continued until work really took over when I was about 35. This importance can be seen in that I had an Olympic trial and also represented the British Universities in two sports, as well as earning half-blues from both Cambridge and Oxford, and full colours from two other universities. And sport also produced a variety of girlfriends!

To my knowledge there was no background of sport in my family. With divorced parents, a father with whom I had no contact, and a mother who because of her smoking could take no exercise, this is not surprising. The only game that I ever played with my mother was French cricket – at which she could last about ten minutes before being exhausted. The problem was compounded by my childhood TB which was not cured until I was nearly eight years old. At Woodford Green Primary School, with the exception of one master, no sport was played, and I have only a vague memory of organised PT. The majority of any games were organised by us in the playground.

And then with my scholarship to Bancroft's School life changed in very many ways, and particularly in sport. In the 1950s sport was important in nearly all public schools. There has been serious criticism of this preponderance over the years but looking back I now realise the advantages both to the pupils and to the community. Competitive sport fosters working within a community, and a wish to be successful – two aspects of life which become very important as one matures. The nonsense of not having examinations from the beginning of schooldays, and with no order of success within a form can only be disastrous for a nation. Some pupils are more clever than others, and some work harder. Very obviously pupils with a less educated background can only reach their full potential with assistance which is essential, but many pupils do markedly improve their own potential by taking part in competitive sport, and long may this occur.

When I started at Bancroft's I was the runt of the form, short and skinny with no muscles. I had good hand eye coordination from somewhere, and I know not where. Over the years I strengthened and improved, but rugby and cricket were still beyond me to really succeed at school. It was not until badminton and athletics were introduced at school that I became competitive. The other attribute that needed no physical prowess, and in which I succeeded from the start was in rifle shooting.

FOURTEEN

SOCCER AND RUGBY

SOCCER

The only time that I have ever played soccer was for my cub team when I was aged about nine or 10. I remember playing as goalkeeper and apart from the one or two local matches for the cubs, I have never played since. I was however taken by my uncle Len to see West Ham United, the team that he supported, on two occasions. But I cannot even remember the scores or who they were playing

Such is my interest in soccer that when I was given a ticket for the semi-finals and the finals of the World Cup in 1966 that England eventually won, I passed the ticket on to one of my colleagues at Surrey University as I had sailing matches on the same days. Had I known that England would be in the final, I would have gone. My only other contact with soccer was meeting Billy Wright, the ex Wolverhampton Wanderer's captain of the team that I had supported as a young boy. Surprisingly this meeting was at Twickenham where he was watching a Varsity match sitting just behind me.

I still occasionally watch soccer on the television, but do feel the acting is now becoming so obvious that it is hardly a sport worth watching at all.

RUGBY

Although suitably equipped with the gear when I went to Bancroft's, without a television at home I had never seen a game of rugby, or even handled a rugby ball. We were to be taught rugby by one of the sons of Lt Col A C Newman VC, an Old Bancroftian. Why the son, although still at school, was not playing himself, I never discovered, but can only assume that there was a medical reason for it. And so we were taught to pass, catch, kick and tackle.

I was definitely not the shape or had the fitness for the game in those early days and was therefore given the position of scrum half. As the years went by I became larger and fitter, and more importantly became a sprinter and moved to be a winger – almost always on the right – but for no obvious reason. Certainly at no point was I near a team until the sixth form when I captained the school third team (Photo 14.1), and played the occasional game for the seconds. In the lower sixth I also started playing for the Old Bancroftians. Third team matches were about one a term, and playing for the Old Boys second team at their ground in Loughton did give me a regular weekly game, and they were obviously short of a winger. And then playing for them I broke my left ankle – and into plaster I went for six weeks. What became obvious to me was that the social side of the game with an excellent and friendly bar was almost as important as the match itself. And the school rule was that anyone who needed to be taken home from the bar was the responsibility of the Old Boys.

In my final year at school I played rugby in the first term and then broke my right wrist (Chapter18), and did not play again until I returned from the Arctic and was at university. And that was for only two or three games for an

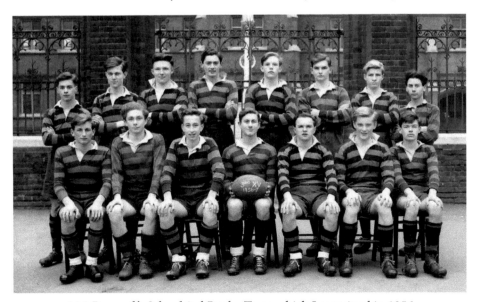

14.1 Bancroft's School 3rd Rugby Team which I captained in 1956

engineering team, partly because I did not really enjoy playing as much as I had done, but more importantly because I was sailing whenever it was possible.

I had thought that these occasional games were my last, but when I was warden of North Side Hall of Residence in London there was an inter hall competition – and my hall was short of a winger. My main memory was that our fly-half was missing tackles all the time, and by the time the ball arrived along their three quarter line I had to make the choice of which of two players to tackle. Luckily I nearly always picked the correct one, and because we had a much stronger pack we did win. Definitely my last game!

Although I was never going to be a competent player I have always enjoyed watching the game. At school it was a requirement that if you were not playing for a team on the Saturday then you were expected to be watching and supporting the school team. When I went to Cambridge I was a regular attender at the Grange Road rugby ground, and particularly if an international team was visiting. It is now an amazing thought in the days of professional rugby that any international team would have a warm up game against the university. And then came Twickenham. Firstly to watch the varsity match, and particularly when my friend and colleague Charles Higham was playing. He was a postgraduate friend in my college, and later a trialist for the England team.

After a gap of many years and with my St John Ambulance hat on, I was for several years on duty as a crowd doctor at internationals at Twickenham. This was interesting and could be quite busy – but nearly always before and after the game and not during (Photo 14.2).

My son-in-law Paul Feenan had been a very keen rugby player at school and at Cambridge, and now my ten year old grandson is performing well. Perhaps my rugby watching days in person rather than on television are not yet over.

There is one large cloud on the horizon of rugby which is the problem of head injuries. Certainly on at least one occasion whilst I was at school I was unconscious for some minutes on the rugby field. I also had more severe head injuries cycling, on the back of a scooter and skiing. A recent MRI scan did show previous damage to my brain. I also well remember what was said about two of the consultants with whom I have worked. They had both been international rugby players, and the comments about them were that they had left their brains on the rugby fields. This problem has now been recognised in rugby, in soccer and in American football, and former players are now suing their clubs for compensation for early dementia. Will the sports continue? A

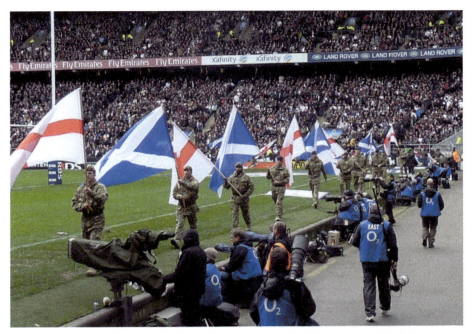

14.2 Twickenham. The Calcutta Cup 2011 at which I was on medical duty.

difficult forecast because the common attitude will be – well it will not happen to me. There have been some changes. Anyone now having a head injury is immediately replaced and has a period off the field before returning for a future game. The only possibilities that I can see for the future is that all players will have to sign away any possible future claims when they start playing, or the rules of the games will have to change. I can see that this is possible in soccer but much more difficult in rugby or American football.

FIFTEEN

CRICKET

A master at Woodford Green Primary School tried to give me an inkling of cricket. I was taken to Lords by a neighbour of ours in Buckhurst Hill when I was aged about 10. It was Peter May's first test match. We sat on the grass at the end opposite to the pavilion. An enormous occasion for a young boy, but apart from the fact that they were playing India I have little other memory. My next visit to Lords was some 55 years later. When I went to Bancroft's School, cricket became an important part of school life during the summer term. The teaching of cricket was not ideal, and in general those of us who had a reasonable ball sense picked it up rather than being well coached, or in fact coached at all.

In the lower forms at school, we travelled nearly a mile each way to the school's extensive playing fields at West Grove, South Woodford. Here the school had some eight pitches. I started life as a fast bowler, and my batting was always somewhat erratic. As I moved up through the school I continued to play, but never at a competitive level until my time in the sixth form when I played for my house team. I was never selected for any of the school teams.

Whilst at Bancroft's I regularly became a scorer for the Woodford Wells cricket team. For this I was paid the princely sum of two shillings and sixpence a week which more than doubled my pocket money. On occasions I was allowed to join them in the nets. Unfortunately I bowled several of them out, and for some reason the invitations ceased. The match that I remember best at Woodford was a Sunday afternoon when Dickie Kent, an Essex player and an

Old Bancroftian, was playing for the Woodford Wells team. He scored more than 160 in his innings, and this was before the days of 20/20 cricket when batting was much more sedate, and to score more than 50 in an afternoon was unusual.

When I went to the University of Leeds, I played the very occasional game, but never at university level. I then went to Cambridge and there the competition to get into a college team was considerably less, and when I did not have a sailing or tennis match I would play cricket at college level. The Department of Chemical Engineering also ran a team that played 20 over cricket on one evening a week. Our team included two people who had played cricket at a senior level. Dr John Turner had won a blue for Cambridge some years previously, and Don Sutherland, a fellow PhD student, was an Australian who had played at junior level for his state team. Our team was very successful and won the league in two consecutive years. I do remember one match when my bowling figures were 8 for 36 – never to be repeated. The other thing about cricket at Cambridge was the fact that in our department as fellow research students we had both an American and a Russian. At nets they came along to try cricket. The American, Hank Schleinitz, was an extremely talented all-round sportsman, playing ice hockey for the University, and had also played baseball in America. Eventually when we were particularly short of players we put Hank into the team. His first ball he hit elegantly towards cover, but then threw his bat down and set off at right angles to the normal running line towards point. We had forgotten to teach him the basic rule of how to score a run. The Russian turned out not to be a success at cricket, but was at least an expert chess player.

When I went as a lecturer to the University of Surrey there was an annual match between the staff and the students. The staff team had two very good players one of whom was a fast bowler, and the other a batsman. By this time I had become a wicket-keeper as my advancing age had slowed my bowling considerably. Amazingly on two succeeding years the staff team beat the student team.

When I returned to Cambridge, I again played for the college on occasions and would open the batting with Roger Knight, who later became captain of the Surrey County team and secretary of the MCC. I always preferred opening the batting as I, both as a batsman and wicket-keeper, much preferred dealing with the fast bowlers than the horrible tweakers. Again the team was reasonably successful, but I was not a regular player because of my other commitments to sailing and to tennis. I do remember however one match when we were playing a team of ex-colonial officers from East Africa. We knew they were rather good, and we had introduced an extra player. He had been a leg break bowler at county level and was now a groundsman to a college. I was the wicket-keeper, and I well remember him telling me to stand up as he started the bowling. The first ball came down at quite a high speed fizzing gently, landed outside the batsman's leg stump and he completely missed it and it hit me. The batsmen turned to me and said that he did not even see the ball, and I replied that neither did I, and it was pure luck that it hit me.

Whilst I was a junior doctor at various hospitals, including in particular in Birmingham we again ran a doctor's team. At Stoke Mandeville Hospital again there was a hospital team which included people both from within the hospital and without. There was also an annual match between the consultants and the rest of the doctors. They would normally beat us, but again we did have one superb South African psychiatrist who had played cricket at national junior level in South Africa. Unfortunately one player was not enough, and we were again beaten. On one occasion one of our plastic surgery juniors was a lady who had played several sports including tennis at close to national level. She was therefore put into the doctor's team to play the rest of the hospital. When she came in, they were very kind to her and bowled relatively slowly. Once they had speeded up the bowling, she had her eye in and there was no stopping her. The slow bowling was a bad mistake as she finished as the highest scorer in our team.. On the occasion of another of our matches one of the plastic surgery consultants, Sanu Desai, who had been a very good cricketer in India was selected. By this stage he was nearly 60 years old, and again playing for the doctor's team against the rest of the hospital, he looked extremely elegant. Unfortunately every stroke was about half to one second late but they still could not get him out.

When I was working at Stoke Mandeville we were living in a small village north of Aylesbury and I played many games for the Whitchurch Cricket Club. I alternated as wicket keeper with Jonathan Freeman-Atwood, a professional classical trumpet player. Several people commented that we were both mad as both our professions required the use of all our fingers. Luckily neither of us was injured.

My last two games of serious cricket were playing for a charity team of surgeons when we were raising money for my research trust. These were being played against a team of Old England test players (Photo 15.1). This had been

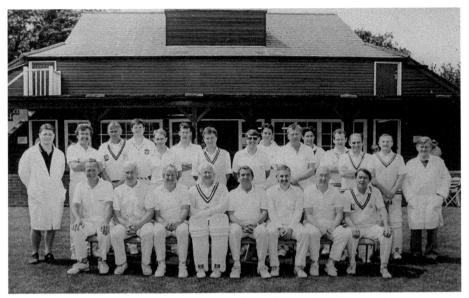

15.1 The Old England cricket team against the Stoke Mandeville research trust team.

arranged for us by Lord Alexander, the President of the MCC, and whose wife was a Vice Patron of the research trust. The first game that we played was at the Rothschild ground just north of Aylesbury. This was a remarkable ground, and the pavilion was a fantastic building listed Grade 1. The captain of their team was Jim Parks, and I believe this was the last game of cricket that he played – having been an extremely successful England wicket-keeper. The second game that we played was at RAF Halton, which was the main ground for the Royal Air Force. I was batting at number 10 and facing the very famous Derek Underwood. We were one run short of tying with Old England and I eventually hit him to mid-wicket and ran as fast as I could. John Lever had picked up the ball at mid-wicket and thrown it at the stumps. Very tragically he hit the stumps spot on when I was about one foot from reaching the other end. I was out and we failed to draw against Old England by one run. What was even more galling was at that time John Lever was the cricket coach at Bancroft's – my old school.

On retirement to the Isle of Wight we had purchased Haseley Manor. Within our grounds was the pitch of the Arreton Cricket Club. Almost needless to say I became involved and over the next fifteen years played the occasional game for them, and also organised teams of friends to play against them. They

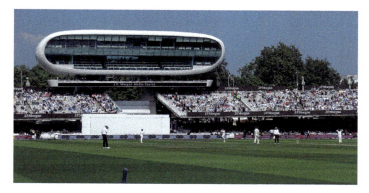

15.2 The media centre at Lords cricket ground.

made me Life President and I still occasionally watch them playing as my right knee no longer permits me to perform.

In recent years I have regularly attended the Lords cricket ground as a doctor for St John working mainly with the crowd, but also with the players when we were required (Photos 15.2 and 15.3). And on one occasion, when they were clearly short of anything to show on the television because of rain showers, they did have pictures of me fielding the ball in my St John uniform. Such is fame. Another memory of Lord's was going to a charity dinner in the Long Room. This had been organised by John Stephenson, the ex-Hampshire captain who was at that time the head of cricket at the MCC – following my old St Caths team mate, Roger Knight. The connection was that his wife was a counsellor for Relate, a charity for whom my wife Vivian was a trustee. The after-dinner speaker was Graham Gooch, and as an Essex man myself it was a great pleasure to meet the famous Graham. He gave the after-dinner speech, and the one joke (or was it) that I remember was his comment about Tuffers, (Phil Tufnell). He said when he was captain of England the great advantage of having Tufnell bowling was the fact that he did not have to think where in the field he was going to put him. Tuffers was not known as a great fielder! I do have the scorecard recording Graham Gooch's famous record-breaking innings of 316, and signed by him at that dinner. And my final memory of Lords was on my last day of St John duty, Dr Tom Evans, the senior St John Lords doctor, had organised for me to receive my St John

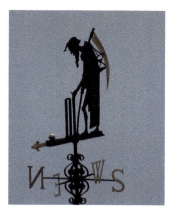

15.3 Old Father Time above the main scoreboard.

Ambulance Long Service Award from the Secretary of the MCC in front of the Pavilion. Both Tom and I were the Royal Protection Group doctors on duty on the occasion of a Royal visit (Photo 15.4).

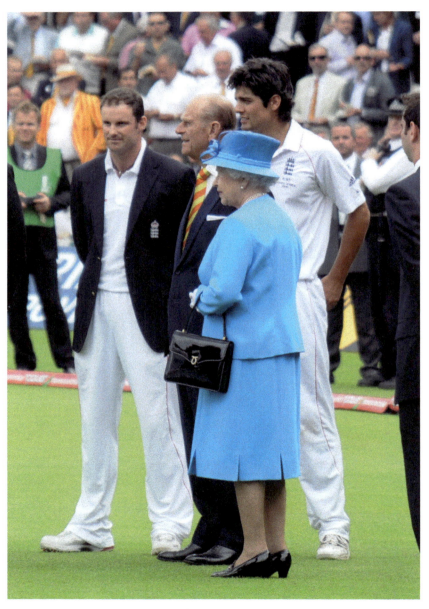

15.4 Her Majesty and the Duke of Edinburgh visiting Lords in 2009. I was on medical duty.

SIXTEEN

BADMINTON, SQUASH AND TENNIS

BADMINTON

Badminton is a strange game. The origins are not at all clear, but it is at least 2000 years old. Again, even where it started is a matter for debate with Greece, China and India all competing for the honour. In the 16th century in England the game was known as battledore and shuttlecock. The battledore was the racket that was used, which was not strung and was a plain piece of wood. It was in those days an upper-class game. The shuttlecock then was already being made with feathers, and this has developed since as plastic is available, but quite unbelievably the feathered shuttlecock is still preferred at the international, national and better club games to the many plastic replacements that, for cost reasons, have been developed. The present shuttlecock weighs approximately 5g, and is made from 16 feathers from either the left-wing or the right-wing of a duck or goose – but not mixed!. These are set into a cork base. They are expensive, and when being played at a high level do not last for very long. Interestingly they have to be humidified for three hours before any game, and at the beginning of every game the players bat about six shuttlecocks until they are all happy with the flight of those that are going to be used in that game. The racket itself weighs some 80 to 90g, so needs considerable strength and flexibility of movement of the wrist especially when playing a clearance from the backhand corner.

Today, badminton is almost 2 separate games. The vast majority of badminton played in Britain is doubles. This is probably because four people can get on to a court, and courts are both expensive and fairly unusual. I understand in the Far East, where it is often the National game, it is played outside with no wind and singles is a much commoner form. But they are very different in other ways as well. Singles needs considerable strength and enormous fitness. It is a defensive game. The smash is unusual. Far commoner is to wish to play from the back of each court with long defensive clearances, and the occasional drop shot making sure that opponents do not stay too far back all the time. From my experience one does indeed need to be fitter to play singles badminton than squash or tennis.

Doubles is a considerably different game. It is far more attacking, and is a game of smash and drop shot with the occasional clearance – again to keep people honest and not crowding at the net. Mixed doubles and either men's or women's doubles are different. In men's or women's doubles the pair tend to play to each side. In mixed doubles the male tends to play at the back, and the female at the front. In fact the male hits far more shots than the female but the speed of reaction of the female is extremely important, as is the ability of the female to do good drop shots.

Except at the highest level in Great Britain, matches tend to be played between three couples on each side. Occasionally a match can consist of three doubles and six singles, but in my experience this is rare.

When I arrived at Bancroft's school in 1950, Badminton was not played. In about my third year, a new chaplain appeared. He was the Rev Dusty Binns (I have no idea what his real Christian name was – but he was known to all the boys in the school as Dusty – and he certainly never stood on his dignity). The Rev Binns was an Anglo-Indian and had lived most of his life in India where he had played badminton at a very high level, and probably as an international. There was a school gymnasium which was of ideal size and height, and the Rev Binns introduced badminton to us when we were in about our fourth year. He was indeed a superb player and instructor. For the whole of our time there, although he was by this stage at least 50 and probably nearer 60 years old he could beat any of us very easily. Badminton was therefore played on one or two evenings each week after school. Several of us became quite proficient and we also started playing matches with the local girls' school, Woodford County High School. I do have memories of these being very important at the time, but I now think that I am too old to remember how important these games with the girls then were. I do not remember any matches with any other boys' school, but I did also begin to play in the local church hall at All Saints Church, Woodford Wells. We must have been progressing well because three of us played in the county junior championship when we were in the sixth form, of whom one reached the semi-final. Unfortunately I had broken my wrist only a few weeks before, and was definitely not at my best with a newly healed right wrist. Again we must have been reasonably proficient because one of us went on to get county colours, and two of us were awarded University colours.

When I went to Leeds, I immediately signed up for the University club, and within a relatively short time was in both the men's doubles team, and the mixed doubles team. In the men's team I had no regular partner, but in the mixed team my regular partner was Dilys Hill. She was a very interesting lady who had qualified as a radiographer before she came to University to read sociology. The other marvellous thing about the mixed doubles team was that the major practice was on a Wednesday evening, and when this finished there was free admission to the university union dance (hop). Not only had Dilys been a radiographer but was also a past gold medal dancer. We played badminton very well together, and after a few months of her instructing me we also danced well together.

When I went on to Cambridge the situation was somewhat different. I immediately started playing badminton for my college, but the University badminton club was only for 30 members who were selected on merit. It took me until my second year before I was asked to join the University club. It was in those days a completely unreal situation. All the members of the University first-team, and half of the second team, were international players. They were not only from Britain but also included players from Singapore, India and Malaysia. The University badminton match was slightly unfair in that Oxford did not have this level of player, and it was regularly a whitewash for Cambridge. I eventually squeezed into the second team on two or three occasions, but certainly I was nowhere near getting a badminton blue.

I then moved to the University of Surrey, which at that time was in Battersea in London, and as with my squash was able to play for the University team. I was immediately selected for the first team, and within a few months was playing in the first pair with a lovely West Indian called Winston. We won several of our matches against other universities. One of our members had played with the Indonesian national team and one year when they arrived in Britain to play in the world championships they came to practice with us. Suddenly a different game.

It was remarkably difficult finding another badminton club with whom to play with other friends in London. Squash and tennis were easy, and the only club that I found in London was that of the university.

When I returned to Cambridge I am delighted to say that my previous membership of the club was sufficient for me to be accepted straightaway into the club. In fact the standard within the University had fallen somewhat, and I had a more regular place in the second team, but again never getting near to the first team. One memory there was when Moira – my then fiancée – was watching me practice with the university club, and afterwards described badminton as the nearest sport to ballet that she had ever seen. Two years later I moved to Oxford, was immediately invited to join the badminton club there, and also instantly had a place in the second team, with the very occasional first team performance. And surprisingly the other thing that I had there, and in fact for the first time in my life, was some formal training by a professional badminton coach. My career in badminton at Oxford was to a large extent truncated. In my second season I spent most of that winter travelling and studying in Africa, and in my third year I spent some 2½ months of the winter travelling and studying in the United States. Knowing the level of the competition for the teams, I think without these long absences I would have certainly been a regular in the second team with a good chance of getting a first-team place and even possibly a blue. But playing against Cambridge then it would certainly have been a losing blue.

After qualifying as a doctor my first house job was at Addenbrooke's Hospital in Cambridge. There I met Chung Hau Oon who had had an astonishing badminton career at international level. After he had played in the world championships in 1969 he became a medical undergraduate at Cambridge. His clinical medicine was at St Mary's Hospital, and they discovered he had one lung full of TB – and he had nearly become All England champion. After a year under treatment he qualified, and his first appointment was as Professor Calne's houseman at Cambridge. I was the best opposition he could find in the hospital and we practised together regularly. He would try out a variety of shots on me which certainly kept me fit, but he would always beat me. Except – one game we were 13 each, and I got a net cord. 14-13. The very next point I got another net cord and although Chung Hau tried very hard he could not return the shot. One game won against a man who had been probably the world number three. I would add that his elder brothers had been world champions. The three brothers were all from Malaysia, and Chung Hau became a cardiologist in Singapore.

The Birmingham Accident Hospital ran a team playing local clubs in Birmingham and I played regularly in that team. I continued to play on occasions for many years. When we moved to the Isle of Wight I still had sufficient ability to be able to play my way into the best club on the Island, but after some months I severely ruptured a muscle in my calf and that was the end of the sport for me.

SQUASH

There were no squash courts at school, and I had neither played nor seen the game when I went to Leeds University. Certainly my priority there was badminton, and it was not until my third or fourth year that I tried a game of squash. The captain of squash gave me some great lessons and we had enjoyable knock arounds.

I did not continue playing squash at Leeds, but when I got to Cambridge, everybody played squash. All colleges would have two or three courts, and it was a very easy game to organise as one only needed one other person, rather than have a whole afternoon or evening devoted to badminton matches. We would in fact very often start to play late in the evenings at nine or 10 o'clock when we left the research laboratory. A quick game then followed by a bath was an ideal way of sleeping well. Having played badminton at a reasonable level, squash was a fairly easy game to learn, and in fact if I'm honest I played badminton on the squash court for the whole of my squash career. This gave me an enormous advantage in playing somebody with whom I had not played before. There is a stroke in badminton called a roundhead smash which does not normally seem to exist in squash. Normally when serving, people would serve from the forehand court toward the backhand side and I was able to do a roundhead smash and put the ball down the line and parallel to the wall, giving me a major advantage.

Within a few months I was playing in the College team, as well as with friends, and continued to do so for the whole of my times in Cambridge. At that time I did not move into the higher echelons of the game. However, when I moved to the University of Surrey as a lecturer, the new university was fairly small, and the lecturing staff regularly played in college teams. I was therefore asked to play in the squash team, and within a few months was the number one in the team. I would say however, that we rarely won against another university.

On one occasion the students challenged the staff to a match. I happened to know that the Bursar's secretary had been the England number two lady squash player when she had been in the Royal Navy. She was in fact an attractive blonde lady, and on seeing her, the captain of the university team was obviously impressed and asked me what number she was going to play. I asked him, "Would you like to play her?" which he did, and very nearly had a major embarrassment. He did eventually beat her 3 games to 2 on fitness rather than ability.

And I did meet my wife playing squash. She was moving to Oxford, and our friend Brian Sweeney gave her my contact details. She went round to my house and we met briefly. I then left her a note asking her if she would like a game of squash which we arranged. She had played squash for her hospital team and was a reasonable player. However the difference between male and female level squash is perhaps more marked than in almost any other game. I realised as we started playing that the only way of making a game of it was for me to play left-handed. A few points later she thought she was doing very well, turned round and saw what I was doing. She did eventually forgive me. Again I was playing with her, and this time we had been playing in a mixed doubles game – always very interesting – with my friends Tony Atkins and Hazel Lishman, a lady radiographer who was a colleague of mine. Some few months later I told Tony that I had just become engaged to one of the people with whom we had been playing squash. His immediate comment.

"Was she the tall thin one or the short fat one." Somewhat of an unfortunate description, but certainly Vivian was not as tall and thin as our radiographer friend. My wife has never forgiven him for giving us a set of scales for our wedding present.

I remember another game when I was in London. I had been recruited as a ringer in a cricket club team and was playing number one. We were in the civil service courts close to Westminster Abbey. As I got on to the court, I noticed my opponent was standing in the backhand court whacking it very hard up and down the backhand wall about 1 inch above the tin. Worrying – and I knew that I was in trouble. Indeed I was, and eventually took only six points off him in the three games. I then asked him.

"Who did you normally play for?" The answer was,

"England." It was indeed the England number two. I then felt somewhat proud of my six points.

At other times I played a couple of other international players. What they would do was to ask two or three capable players to practice. They would then stay on the court whilst we would rotate every second or third game. This was extremely good for their fitness training, very useful for us, and after a few rotations we would occasionally start to win the odd game.

Another game that I remember well was when I went to teach anatomy in the University of Zambia. One of the basic ways of amusement in Zambia and throughout southern Africa was sport. A local player therefore challenged me to a game of squash, and to my surprise, against a not very good player, I lost. I had never played at four thousand feet before and the altitude had a very marked effect. About two weeks later the same man would rarely get a point off me.

And then the final game of my serious squash career. By this stage I was married, and we and the family were on our way to Australia. Our first step was to stay with Brian and Jenny Sweeney in the Philippines. Brian had been a very good friend of mine in Cambridge where we had played squash on many occasions – and of course he had introduced me to Vivian. We arrived in Manila after a very long journey and late, after an even longer than the usual journey by plane from Bangkok to Manila which had gone wrong, and had had to return. We therefore got off the plane in Manila after some 18 or 20 hours all very exhausted. The temperature was 99°F, the humidity 99%. Brian welcomed me with open arms, and said how glad he was that we had arrived.

"You are playing squash tonight in the match of the year." This was the Australians in the Philippines against the English in the Philippines. When I got to the court which had no air-conditioning I looked around totally aghast, then had the brilliant idea of approaching the eldest of the Australians, and suggesting that we played the best-of-three rather than the best-of-five. Luckily he fell for it, and I beat him 9-0, 9-1. Had it gone one more point I would have been dead. And so a very pleasant memory to finish my squash career.

TENNIS

It was unfortunate that there were no tennis courts at Bancroft's School, particularly as the two brothers of Christine Truman were, the Wimbledon ladies losing finalist of 1958. They were some years above me at school and had both played at Wimbledon. There was also Martin Braund in my year, and he was Christine's mixed doubles partner at Wimbledon, and also the losing semi-finalist in the Junior Wimbledon championships of 1957. Keith Noakes, who was also in my year, was my introduction to tennis and we started playing occasionally on park courts in Ilford when we were in the fifth form. I did play once with Christine, and in fact many years later went out with her younger sister Nell when she was at Oxford. When I got to Leeds University I started playing more. This was men's doubles and mixed tennis. An excellent way of meeting young ladies, and I progressed sufficiently to play both for Devonshire Hall, within which was a Junior Wimbledon player, and for the university second team on two occasions.

And then to Cambridge where I played regularly for my college, St Catharine's, and with several friends both male and female. As I have said before it was an excellent way of meeting the opposite sex and I well remember the Milner twin sisters, Jo and Sue, who had come up from London, and also Liz Weech. One game that I also remember was playing with Helen Dreesmann. Helen was a daughter of one of the owners of the well known stores Vroom and Dreesman which was the Dutch equivalent of Marks and Spencers. She was at the Bell School of languages which was the best known of the Cambridge language schools. We had met at a party as the girlfriend of one of my flatmates was teaching at school. After the game I was asking Helen where she was staying in Cambridge. Her answer was one of the classics of all time.

"I am staying with a retarded colonel and his wife."

After Cambridge came London. At the University of Surrey I played on many lunch breaks with a regular four in Battersea Park and elsewhere whenever there was an opportunity. On one of these occasions my good friend Dubbie Smith asked me to make up a four with a girl that I had not met before – Moira Megaw. Within a few weeks we were engaged. I continued to play for my college teams when I returned to Cambridge and in Oxford. Between these I spent the summer working in Zambia and played regularly. That was a new experience in that it was a requirement of the club that one employed local lads as ball-boys. As soon as a point was finished a new ball was thrown to you, and the loss of a minute to collect a ball and the altitude I still remember being exhausted.

I later played occasionally with Vivian, my fiancée and later wife, when we played in Birmingham and regularly in Australia during our year living there. We have continued playing regularly until my knee gave out about five years ago. Among the places that we have played were our own grass court in Aston Abbotts, and in our present house where we have an outdoor asphalt court, and also the only indoor court on the Island. What else can you do with a large unused barn?

My other tennis involvement has been with St John Ambulance at Wimbledon which I did on a regular basis for fifteen years. It could be a surprisingly busy duty as Court 1 was open to the sun and people in the stands could stand up after severe sun exposure, collapse and fall down several layers of stairs. There were also the normal variety of problems coming into the three units, and there was a small area where I could do minor surgery under local anaesthetic. For some years we were privileged as doctors to stand in the entrance area for the players and I saw several of them. What surprised me was that nearly all the lady players were taller than me – and I am 5' 10". The four or five doctors were also given a centre court ticket and so we would normally see some of the action unless too busy (Photo 16.1).

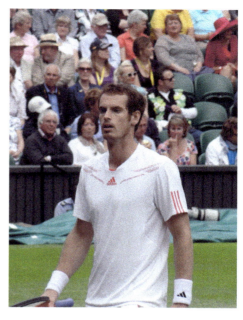

16.1 Andy Murray playing in the men's singles at Wimbledon 2012. I was on medical duty.

SEVENTEEN

SWIMMING, SCUBA DIVING, CANOEING AND ROWING

SWIMMING

I have no memories of going into water except for my regular baths until I was about 10 or 11. My first ventures into a swimming pool were with the cubs at Walthamstow Baths. This was in fact paddling in the shallow end and certainly I was unable to swim. I was still not swimming when I went to Bancroft's where there was a small indoor swimming pool 17 yards long by 17 feet wide. It was not heated and swimming was a summer sport and in gymnastics time. I was still struggling to have the confidence to be able to get out of my depth, but to pass a scout test for my second class badge I had to be able to swim 100 yards. At school, I eventually managed to swim one width still in my depth at which point the gym master, Mr Wright, told me to get in the deep end and swim towards the shallow end. I survived this and ever after wondered what had been the problem. There was one other interesting occurrence at school in that Mr Wright said to everybody that they did not need to worry about being out of their depth, because everybody could float. At which point Ian Williams in my form and I both took a deep breath and sat on the bottom of the pool. Certainly there was no talk again about the ability to float. I continued to swim both at school, and at Walthamstow and my prowess continued to improve slowly. It turned out I was far better at backstroke than either breast stroke or crawl. Diving in any form I was certainly not keen on, and perhaps this explained why I was better at backstroke, as the race started in the water without needing to dive.

There were of course inter house yearly swimming competitions. Mr Wright, the gym master, had a clever way of making sure that we all took part. Clearly I was not going to win any race in the water, but each boy who swam 50 lengths of the bath (almost half a mile) each year scored one point for his house. The time did not matter.

As I was progressing up the school, I was also progressing up my scout badge ladder towards my Queen's Scout badge. To obtain the Queen's Scout badge one needed first aid, the seaman's badge, and two other badges of a public service variety. One of the badges that I took was the lifesaving badge. I cannot remember the full details now but it did include swimming in clothes, undressing in the water and also rescuing somebody in the water and then getting them out of the swimming bath. Having obtained this badge I discovered that the National Lifesaving badge at the basic level was very similar, and I therefore added this to my growing collection of badges.

Amazingly my other swimming exploit was to win a backstroke race. It was at the Scout jamboree in Sweden in 1956, and I was volunteered to represent the British team in the backstroke. Swimming in the Baltic Sea was extremely cold, but the weather was sunny and one could see the finishing line, which looked about 200 yards away. I therefore set off at a suitable speed and kept my position at the front of the international teams. 200 yards on a sunny beautiful day was a vast underestimate of the actual distance. I did however manage to finish and won my first and only swimming prize. It was interesting that the competition at both breaststroke and at crawl was extremely intense. It appears that the backstroke was not a form of swimming that many other countries practised.

Swimming was a necessity for sailing dinghies. If one was a competent swimmer in decent weather one did not wear a lifejacket, certainly on inland waters. I am pleased to say that I never needed my swimming ability whilst sailing, as although I capsized many times at no point did I ever lose contact with the boat.

My other swimming story of that vintage was whilst I was a student in Devonshire Hall at the University of Leeds. There was an interhall competition, in which I had no part. However in Devonshire there was an excellent student swimmer who represented the University at several distances. The weekend of the interhall competition was when his younger brother, still at school, was visiting. Also an excellent swimmer, and we put him in the team as a ringer. Unfortunately he broke two University records and we were disqualified.

When I was living in London between 1964 and 1967 a group of us would ice skate in the winter and go swimming in the Chelsea Mansions swimming pool in the summer. This was certainly not serious swimming, until my then girlfriend Moira joined us. She was a brilliant swimmer, and had actually been asked to train for the British Olympic diving team. Needless to say none of us could keep up with her, and the only time that I ever beat her was when, as might be expected, we were swimming backstroke.

And since then I have always disliked swimming in England and even in the south of Australia, as I have found the water always to be too cold. This of course was before the days of wetsuits. The only times that I regretted not being able to swim were in Africa, firstly when I was teaching anatomy in Zambia. One did not swim in Africa in still water because of the risk of bilharzia – then incurable. On my way home I had two days in Dar es Salaam and there in the heat and the sunshine the sea looked extremely inviting. I therefore swam slowly out, but after about 10 minutes the thought of sharks entered into my somewhat addled brain. I swam back to the beach far more rapidly than I had swum out.

My second swimming story was again in Africa. During my medical elective in Zululand most of the doctors in the hospital arranged to have a weekend at the famous Rorke's Drift. Again bilharzia had been a worry during my time, but the Buffalo (Mzinyathi) River at Rorke's Drift was flowing sufficiently fast that the snails which carry the disease were not present. Just above the drift itself there was a large lake approximately one hundred and fifty yards in diameter. I thought this looked awfully inviting on a perfect day, and having swum about two thirds across the lake suddenly realised that it wasn't as still as it had looked and I was being quite rapidly swept towards the waterfall at the end of the lake. I accelerated and got to the other side in time. I could understand why several of the soldiers fleeing from the battle of Isandlwana had drowned at Rorke's drift in 1879. That had been in the rainy season when the river would have been flowing much more rapidly.

I have hardly been in the water to swim since then.

SCUBA DIVING

At Seaview on the Isle of Wight in 1962 or 1963 my best friend at the time was Barry Hook (later Barry Stobart-Hook). He was competent at many things, and this included scuba-diving. He thought I should have a go at it, but unfortunately he had only one set of gear. I put on this gear with the admonition in my ear that if the bubbles stopped coming up he would come down and get me. It was cold, I could see about 2 foot in front of my nose and having dived for about one minute decided that I had had enough of scuba-diving. And that was the end of my scuba diving career.

CANOEING/KAYAKING

Canoeing comes in two forms. Kayaking or Canadian canoeing. Both forms I tried with the Scouts. My first canoeing trip was to Denmark for our Scout summer camp in 1954 or 1955, when in Canadian canoes we canoed down the Gudena river. Towards the origin of the river there were various minor rapids at which points we picked up the canoes and walked along the bank until the water became suitably deep enough to continue canoeing. Every night we camped in a local farmer's field, and all our gear was of course in the canoes with two people in each canoe. I am delighted to say that we were the only crew that did not capsise. There was however one interesting night where we had reached the wider part of the river and had been canoeing for several hours and were suitably tired. It had been a pretty foul day with rain and no sign of sun, and we came across this beautiful area of grass with the river looping around it. We asked the local farmer, who looked at us rather strangely, and gave us permission to camp. It was a superb campsite until about 3 o'clock in the morning, when the rain of that day caused the river level to rise. The farmer's wife came out to rescue us, saw the problem and invited as all into a barn with hot tea provided. She then cooked a lovely breakfast for which we were very grateful. The rest of the holiday passed without incident.

I have only once kayaked competitively in my life. Again the scouts – there was an Essex Scout competition for two-man kayaking along the River Crouch in Essex. I teamed up with Michael Verlander who was minimally younger than I was, but about twice my size, and certainly twice my strength. For his later National Service he served as a Marine Commando. It was meant to be a 10 mile race down the Crouch, finishing up at the Royal Burnham Yacht Club. There was however a strong spring tide flowing in, and we worked out afterwards that we actually kayaked some 13 miles. Michael and I had had no previous experience, and certainly no training. I still have memories towards the end of the race of being completely tired out from the impossible task and that I would have been very happy to have capsized and drowned. We finished, and unbelievably out of about 40 troops competing, mostly well trained, we came third. Never again.

ROWING

I had pottered about in small rowing boats with the scouts at Maylandsea Bay Sailing Club and was at least safe at sea. The one occasion there that I well remember was a day when the wind was blowing a full gale and no one was sailing. A man then launched his Class11+ dinghy, put up the sails and lasted about one minute. He tried several times to right it unsuccessfully and two of us rowed out to help.

"If you take the sails down before righting it you have a much better chance," was our advice. This he did, and we towed him in. His comment afterwards was,

"Sailing is not as easy as driving a London bus!" – his normal occupation. It was his first ever sail and the lack of other boats on the water had by-passed him.

When I went to Cambridge in 1961 I, as most men do, decided to try rowing on the Cam. The research students of the Department of Chemical Engineering decided to make up an eight. Because we were from a collection of colleges we could not compete in the inter-college bump races and therefore arranged to join the Association of Cambridge University Assistants (ACUA) races. We needed a coach, and somebody recruited the Rev Bailey Jones. Jellybones as he was known was the Dean of Trinity College, an old Oxford rowing blue and a marvellous character – the ideal coach. I took my place near the bows, and Suman Das, a six stone Indian and a brilliant academic, but not in the same league as a sportsman, was the cox. Unfortunately as we set off Suman kept pulling the wrong string and we went from bank to bank with Jellybones yelling,

"Hold hard," at regular intervals. After a few minutes he looked at me who he had somehow discovered was a sailor, and Suman and I were ordered to change places. And that was the last time that I rowed. I became a cox although at 10st 3lbs somewhat heavy. In both Oxford and Cambridge if a boat makes a bump on each of the four days of the races every member of the crew can buy

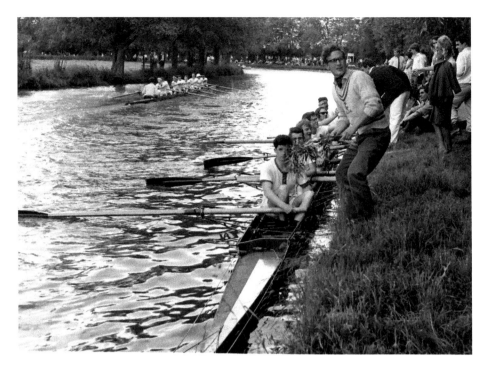

17.1 St Catherine's college Cambridge graduate boat winning oars 1963.

a beautifully painted oar. The cox only got a painted rudder which are at least easier to display. I still have my first rudder after success in the ACUA races. The next races for which I was recruited was the College IVth boat, rowed by graduates (Photo 17.1). Another rudder. This was followed by a rugby crew boat as their cox had become ill a few days before the bump races a year later. Another rudder. I took part in two more series of bump races, but we failed to win our oars again.

When I moved to Oxford the home of the medical students was Osler House (later Green Templeton College). We were admitted as a College to the races, but had to start at the bottom of all of the divisions. The way it worked was that every time a boat made a bump, on the next day of the four it changed places at the start with the bumped boat. This meant that any boat could only move up four places in any one year. I was recruited to cox for the practising, but was overseas for the races. A pity as earning oars was a formality as we had two former blue oarsmen, and several others with considerable experience in the boat.

Coxing in normal races on a straight course must be extremely boring. Coxing on the Cam and on the Isis is much more interesting and requires considerable skill to travel the shortest distance using as little rudder as possible, as that slows the boat. My various boats decided that even with my weight I was suitably skilled, In total I made nineteen bumps or overbumps, and was never bumped. An unusual record.

My final competitive race was at Sea View Yacht Club when I was the Assistant Secretary. Seaview as a village has Summer sports on and in the water. This includes rowing, swimming, walking the greasy pole and various other challenges. One of the races is the Rescue Race. Each team is two people. The one swimming sets off from the shore, and the one rowing (a pram dinghy) sets off from a line way out at sea when the gun goes. They meet, the swimmer climbs aboard, and the oarsman then sets off back to the finishing line out at sea from where they started. Two brilliant swimmers in the club were the Bonhams' – mother and daughter. I was paired up with daughter Eve and we won easily.

EIGHTEEN

ATHLETICS

When I went to Bancroft's only three sports were really organised. Rugby in the first term, hockey in the second, and cricket in the summer term. The PT (physical training) master was Sgt Major West – an ex-paratrooper who was responsible for the two PT lessons a week which could include the swimming pool. He also organised occasional cross country runs. With no previous experience these runs suited me and I would normally come within the first three or four in my year. Runs in the London clay of Epping Forest were a challenge and particularly when it was wet, muddy and cold in the winter months. And then one foul day when running through a wet and very muddy stream I lost a plimsoll. Despite a long search it was well buried and I could not find it and had to walk/hop back to school. That put me off cross country running, certainly in the Forest, and from which I never properly recovered. One thing that one learned very rapidly was not to come to school with a note from home saying one had a cold or similar and one was not well, Sgt Major West's instant response was to say that you were excused gym and the best way of improving a cold was to go for a run – and off one was sent for a thirty minute run in the Forest. Sick notes ceased to appear very rapidly.

Some four years later the Reverend Binns became the school chaplain. 'Dusty' Binns as he was instantly called was an Anglo-Indian who had played badminton at international level for India and rapidly introduced the game to the school (Chapter 16). Almost at the same time Mr Wright, a properly trained sports master, appeared and he introduced athletics into the Spring term programme alongside the hockey. A grass running track was set up and the very scruffy jump pit cleaned up. It became apparent that even with no training I was a very competent sprinter, could long jump and triple jump and throw the javelin. What I could not do was the high jump or the high hurdles. I was still very short at that time. Nor could I afford spiked running shoes.

In my lower sixth year I sprinted in both 100yd and the 220yd races, and was persuaded to try a 440yd race. Very unsuccessful, but far worse was a 440yd hurdle race where I finished the last few yards almost walking. That summer I competed in a national scout athletic meeting in the 100yds race. I had borrowed a set of spikes, and it was the first time that I had run on a cinder trap. As I was preparing for the start I noticed the lad on my right was watching his trainer fix and adjust a pair of starting blocks – something which I did not have, and had never used. I was beaten by several yards. The lad was Colin Frith – the national junior champion and record holder. I did come second in 10.0 seconds and still have a certificate presented to me by Harold Abrahams the 1924 Olympic 100m gold medallist made famous in the film 'Chariots of Fire'.

In my upper sixth year Mr Wright also introduced pole vaulting. It was then very different to today. The poles were solid and non-flexible, originally of bamboo, and then an aluminium pole was obtained. The other major difference was that one landed in sand and not absorbent sponge. This required that one landed on one's feet or it was fairly painful, especially if the sand was wet. Several of us tried it. One lad two years above me did exceptionally well at just over 11', and this was sufficient to be the fourth best junior in Britain at the time. My best height was 9' 6" – and then disaster. On one jump I caught the bar on my wrist and when I landed, not on my feet, I sat on the bar and there was a nasty, and very painful, crack. Even worse was that it was my wrist and not the pole that was broken. I had been practising with my very good friend Roger Whiteley and it was he and not me that very nearly fainted. Off to Whipps Cross Hospital I was taken. The hospital phoned my mother and the message that she heard was that I was in casualty, and had been revolting! Having sorted out what had actually happened to me she came to see me and after an X-ray which showed fractures of the radius, ulna and scaphoid of my right wrist it was manipulated and plastered under an anaesthetic. I returned for a check-up the following day when a further anaesthetic and re-setting was necessary.

Mr Wright is almost certainly long dead, and regrettably I never did thank him for the marvellous advice that he gave me when I was fifteen.

"If you want to be a serious athlete, give up smoking now!"

At that time I had been stealing my mother's cigarettes since the age of nine or ten and smoking them on the way home from cubs or scouts. I have always been grateful that I took his advice, although I failed to become an Olympic athlete.

That summer I was on the expedition to Finnish Lapland with a somewhat weak wrist which had just come out of plaster, but survived without any problems. And then to Leeds University in September. I considered doing athletics as my main sport but knew that my wrist was not yet ready for pole vaulting. A pity as the university record was 6" lower than my school height. Instead sailing became my main sport.

Ten years later when I returned to Cambridge as a medical student I must unfortunately have been talking about my former brilliant athletic career. Athletic cuppers (the inter college championship) was in a few weeks' time, and my college did not have a pole-vaulter. I had little option but to borrow some spikes and with no practice for ten years came third out of six, and I also ran the 100ms.

A few months later a thirty mile charity walk was organised. I entered and started trying to collect donations from friends. The almost universal response was that if I ran it, they would back me. With no option and absolutely no training I, and about 200 of the 10,000 people taking part did indeed run. Amazingly I came in the top ten! I was so exhausted that I had trouble cycling back to my digs, and I needed the next couple of weeks to fully recover.

Many years later I nearly had to do a marathon. When I set up my medical research charity in the 1980s one of the original trustees was Gavin Campbell of 'That's Life' fame whom I had met when I was the medical adviser to the programme. Gavin said that the next year he was going to do the London marathon – and so was I! Unfortunately – or possibly fortunately – he was injured, and I have never done a marathon.

NINETEEN

ICE HOCKEY AND FIELD HOCKEY

ICE HOCKEY

As a young teenager it was possible to walk on the ice which formed on the lakes in Epping Forest during most winters. At one scout jumble sale there was a pair of ice skates on offer for 5 shillings (25p). They were less than ideal as they strapped on shoes or ideally boots – but my army boots were ideal. I started skating and fairly rapidly was not falling over. The person on the ice who surprised me was my GP, Dr Grogono who must have been nearly fifty and was skilfully figure skating. He said hello but did not offer me any lessons. Another pair of skates with flat blades appeared at a later jumble sale which included the boots – and those I also bought.

Ice skates are of three basic types. Figure skates have a slightly rounded base and some barbs at the front for spinning, jumping etc. Hockey skates have a flat profile and no barbs, and the blades are close to the length of the boot. Racing skates also have a flat profile but are nearly twice as long as the boot.

I skated occasionally on ponds when I was at Leeds but never on a rink, and then off to Cambridge where I was for the famous winter of 1962/63 – the 'Big Freeze'. It was cold. −26°C was recorded in Cambridge. In my large room in college I recorded −20°C, and with the heating – a shilling in the slot gas fire – full on, it was −10°C. One slept in pyjamas, and then in a sleeping bag within the normal bed clothes. The loos were freezing up throughout the college and our one did not freeze as it was being used every five minutes throughout the night when it was almost the last one working.

One of the marvellous memories of my life was skating with some friends on a moonlit night on the ice on a fen just outside the city. There was no wind and a full moon, and the sound of the skates stays with me still. The next thing that happened was chance. I was sharing a house with an American and two Canadian fellow research students. The American, Hank Schleinitz, and one of the Canadians, Bob Perz, were already playing in the university ice hockey team and they suggested that I should try the game which was being played on the frozen River Cam between St John's College and Trinity College bridges. It was an ideal piece of ice with a high wall on one side, and a lower wall on the other. And so with a borrowed stick and padding and my old skates I played for one or two hours every day for the next four or five weeks. There were occasional snow falls which had to be cleared, but the night skies were normally moonlit, and the ice remained for the whole of that term. By this stage I was converted and joined the club.

The history of ice hockey is interesting. It is thought to have started in Canada, possibly by British military personnel who were stationed there in the late 18th century. Certainly it was being played outside in the 1800s, and the first indoor match was in Montreal in March 1875. Incredibly the first match which is still in existence today was between Oxford and Cambridge Universities at St Moritz in 1885. Surprisingly an ice hockey competition was held in the *Summer* Olympics of 1920, and then moved to the Winter games in 1924. In 1936 the British team were the gold medallists. And then came the war and afterwards the game became much less popular in Britain, with many rinks closing to the game in the 50s and 60s. There was a resurgence in the 70s and 80s and it is now played enthusiastically throughout the country, and by both male and female teams. It became for women an Olympic sport in 1998. A team consists of a maximum of fifteen players. It is made up of three attack lines of three, two defence lines of two and two net minders. What are in effect the reserve lines of both attack and defence are the least skilled and are often on the ice for short periods only unless one team is way ahead. This situation was marked at both Oxford and Cambridge in that in the fifies and early sixties only eleven half blues were awarded to each team. This had occurred since 1933 when the first half blues were awarded at the time that the match was moved from Europe to England. I am pleased to say this changed to all fifteen players being half blues in the late sixties. Up until then only six sports had been awarded full blues but this changed in all sports in 2016 when discretionary full blues could be awarded for those who were at, or close to, international standard.

The river did not freeze sufficiently to skate for the next few years, and as there was then no ice rink in Cambridge, and apart from some skill training in a gym, we had to travel either to Brighton or to Birmingham to practice. We would leave in a coach at about 6pm to arrive when normal skating had finished at 10pm. After two hours of skating we then set off back to Cambridge. The coach driver certainly thought that he was Stirling Moss, and the drive could be quite exciting. We arrived back at about 2.30am and then at work or in a lecture for nine-o-clock.

I practiced with the team for the next year, and then played as one of the three extras in the occasional game. I always remember the first of these matches. The whole team went into a huddle and the captain started encouraging us forcibly to be really vicious and not give in. Very American, and totally different to anything in which I had been involved in other sports. The pre-game huddle now seems to have spread to Britain in many sports! It was an unfortunate time when rinks were closing for ice hockey as many of them were taken over by a company, Silver Blades, who thought ice hockey players were a nasty rough bunch. And so Streatham and Richmond were two rinks where we played the last game for many years. I did play at Wembley and also against Brighton Tigers – the best team in England at the time. At that time we were considered wimps as we were the only team who all wore helmets. Even with my helmet I unfortunately finished that game with a broken nose and a minor head injury which meant that I took part in the European tour which followed with a plaster on my nose. I was extremely lucky to have been selected for that British Universities tour to Austria and Italy which was made up almost totally of players from the Oxford and Cambridge clubs. If I am honest it was probably that a driver for a mini-coach was required. But I did play in the Innsbruck Olympic stadium where we lost 6 – 5 to what was in effect the Austrian national team. We had some exceptional players, and especially Davey Johnston who had previously captained the American students team. What was in effect the British Universities team had only three Englishmen, and one of us was Richard Fidler who had been raised in Canada when his father was stationed there as a diplomat. The rest of the team were Canadian, American and one each from Russia and Norway. With that amount of skilled players I was on the ice for about two minutes. Some of the other teams that

ICE HOCKEY AND FIELD HOCKEY

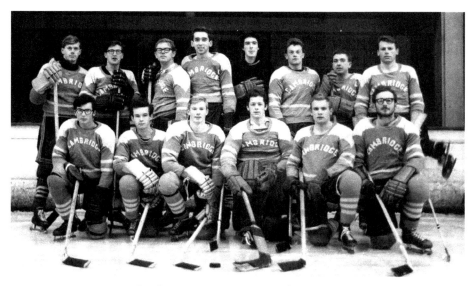

19.1 Cambrige University Ice Hockey Team 1968

we played were Kitzbuhel, Saas Fe and Zell am Zee and in Italy the two teams were less of a challenge and I had a little more ice time.

The first of my Blues matches (Oxford vs Cambridge) was in my last year. I played, but not being selected as one of the best eleven players, did not get my half blue (Photo 19.1).

After I left and moved to London I continued to practice with the team, and also played the occasional game for the London Ambassadors and the Birmingham Barons – for which I was paid! I was also skating regularly with friends at the Queen's Club – where hockey skates were banned, and at Richmond who were more enlightened.

And then in 1967 I returned to Cambridge and immediately started playing seriously again. The quality of our team was of a lower standard than three years previously and I was in the second attack line and was therefore awarded my half blue – a sweater that I still wear with pride. It also meant that I was eligible to be elected to the Hawks Club for which a full blue or more than one half blue was required. One half blue and two sports at British Universities level was sufficient. A second British Universities tour to Austria was organised. Again Oxford, Cambridge and London players made up the team. I was appointed captain – and I am certain that was because I was the only Brit in the team. An interesting tour but considerably less successful.

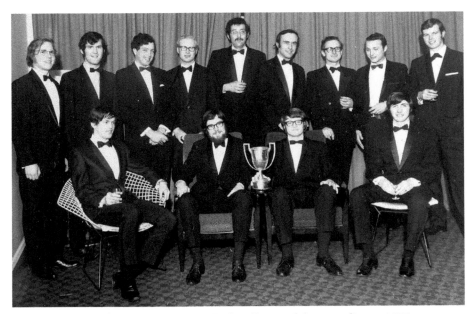

19.2 Oxford University Ice Hockey Team celebratory dinner 1970.

There were some interesting players at that time. Our net minder was also the University cricket wicket keeper. He was South African and not a brilliant skater but a man with amazing reflexes. The reserve net minder was Martin Kubelik, a son of the famous Czechoslovakian classical music conductor. One memory of Martin was that his car had studded ice tyres which were illegal in the UK, but the performance on icy roads was unbelievable. Another of our team was a Canadian Roman Catholic priest. Great on the ice with his red hair and fiery temper. The marvellous memory of the Father was the look on his face when the announcer broadcast,

"Two minutes in the sin bin for dirty play for Father Mc Candless."

In 1969 I moved to Oxford, and made a bad mistake. Having played for Cambridge the year before, playing for Oxford made me the player to get – and they did. I spent more time flat on the ice than in any other game in my career. We did however win 3 – 2, and I did score the winning goal (Photo 19.2). As I was overseas for the next two varsity matches that was almost the end of my ice hockey career. I did mention in Chapter 8 that I played one game at the University of Michigan, and to my surprise, and for the only time in my life, I was the best player on the ice.

A marvellous sport.

FIELD HOCKEY

Hockey was the school game for the spring term. It needed less muscles and bulk than the rugby of the previous term, and as the runt of the year I enjoyed it far more. I was happier playing on the right wing, and continued to do so for the succeeding three years. In my fourth year I was playing in the school under 15s team, but half way through the year was displaced by Roger Furness from the year below me. I forgave him three years later when he was awarded his first England cap.

I did not play at all at Leeds University. Cambridge (and Oxford) are different. There were only a few hundred undergraduates in any college, and all colleges ran one or more teams for every sport. Players had to be found, and anyone who played any sport was recruited. Two good friends Brian Robson and David Groom, both university first team players were after me, and I was recruited. By this time I had not played hockey for six years and had been playing ice hockey. Unfortunately they forgot to remind me of the rules. The first player from the opposition came dribbling down the touch line and I put a very effective hip into him and watched happily as he finished up in a large heap. For some reason the umpire was definitely not impressed, but partly forgave me when I explained the problem. I did play once or twice again at Cambridge.

When I was a junior doctor back at Cambridge, this time at Addenbrooke's Hospital, the doctors ran a mixed hockey team. A very different and much more dangerous game for a man. The ladies whom we were playing were distinctly vicious, and we were trying to be gentlemen. We did have an ex British international and an ex Kenyan player in the team, and were never beaten. The British player was the more amazing. He must have been over sixty years old, played at full back and hardly moved – but nobody went past him. And that was the end of my field hockey career.

TWENTY

SKIING

Skiing was always one of those things that I had wished to do, but had not had the opportunity or the money.

On my first ice hockey tour of the continent in 1963/64, I had arranged to meet Berbel Mattka, a German lady that I had met at Seaview when she was visiting the Birchenough family for whom she had previously worked as a nanny. She was with a party of German friends, one of whom was clearly her new boyfriend. They were all expert skiers and after a brief lunch disappeared up the mountain at high speed. I had the opportunity to hire a set of skis to try it out. The skis were wooden, truly antique, with ancient bindings of the bear trap type. I found a suitable flat piece of snow, put on the very old boots and skis and started to try to walk. I remember it being very different to walking with skates. I eventually found a slight slope and needless to say managed to fall over fairly rapidly. After about half an hour I had progressed a few yards without falling over and was learning to turn. Skiing is completely different to ice skating. On skis one leans out to turn – in ice hockey you lean in. In fact the only thing that is the same between the two is the crash stop, the one thing that I could do automatically with my ice hockey background. I had no further chance to try skiing on that trip as we were playing hockey in a different town or village each night and travelling between them during the days.

And so it was about two years later at the age of 28 when I had saved up enough money to go skiing, I joined some friends for a trip to Zermatt with Murison Small and stayed in one of their chalets. We arrived on the Saturday evening, and the next day I hired a somewhat more modern pair of boots and skis and had the Sunday to practice on these with help and encouragement from the friends before joining a class on the Monday morning. Zermatt is an interesting and very beautiful ski resort, but less than ideal for beginners as the nursery slopes are actually relatively steep. One got up to these slopes in the small mountain railway. Having got off the train I could see the ski school about 200 yards below. I therefore put on my new skis and gently skied down to them, arriving with a crash stop. I asked for class I and the instructor in charge immediately said that if you can stop like that you are in class 2. The fastest promotion I have ever had. In fact it turned out to be an appropriate class. I think all of the people had had prior experience, but none of them were very good or very confident or very fit. I at least was very fit, and almost certainly overconfident after my one day of skiing. However by the end of the second or third day I was keeping up very easily and towards the end of the week was as competent, and probably more so than anyone else in the class. The one person I remember was a somewhat overweight gentleman who was certainly not competent but great fun. He would happily ski down the nursery slope at high-speed until crashing on every occasion. Arising from the cloud of snow created came a few rude words – much to the amusement of the rest of the class and I think of him also.

Class 2 finished on the Friday and I therefore had a weekend with the other people in our chalet. This included Meg Proud, my girlfriend with whom I had signed up for the trip. I therefore spent those two days again practising very hard indeed. On the Monday what had been my class 2 was to become class 3. I felt confident my skiing was slightly above the level that the class had reached and therefore joined a class 4. There was a delightful ski instructor called Eddie Aufdenblatten. He obviously believed in keeping his class to a size of only 10 people and so if somebody else came along looking for class 4 he would say,

"Are you looking for a starting class 4 or a senior class 4?" If they said starting class 4 he would point them down to another class 4 just down the slope. If they said they wanted a senior class 4 he pointed them to the same class – to which they happily skied.

It was indeed a good class 4, and certainly I was the least capable in the class, perhaps not surprising after only one week. Again my fitness helped enormously, and I was just about able to keep up. At the end of the day Eddie said that I could come back the next day, but if by the end of the second day I was still holding everybody up I would be demoted. In fact on the second day I did keep up and as we were finishing the lesson on that day, he came up to me and the other young male student who was in the class, and asked if we would like to ski down to the village with him. Silly question! We therefore had a marvellous and free private lesson. In fact not quite free as we had to buy Eddie a drink or two when we arrived back into the village. And this continued for the rest of the week. Eddie was by far the best instructor I came across in my skiing career. His job during the summer was working as a builder, but clearly skiing and teaching skiing were his favourite pastimes.

And then on the final day, I challenged Meg to a race. I would say that Meg had skied for some four or five years prior to this trip, and was extremely able and fit. One of the other members of our group acted as the umpire. I was sent off 30 seconds before Meg and just before reaching the finishing line was passed by the umpire himself going flat out to catch me. It turned out that I had won easily as Meg had fallen over just after the start. It was a holiday not to be forgotten, and at the end of it I was totally committed to skiing.

Skiing is a strange sport. There are two types, downhill skiing which was my interest, and langlaufing which is done on longer skis and basically on the flat with gentle climbs up and skiing down – and hard work! One of the problems which is more obvious with downhill skiing is the dependence on the weather conditions. One occasionally has the perfect day, when the sun is shining, the snow is newly fallen – ideally on the previous night – there is no strong wind blowing and the slopes are almost empty from other people. Rare occasions. Far more commonly it is cold, windy, the snow is icy and there are crowds.

On returning to the University of Surrey several things happened which made skiing the next year impossible. Firstly I became engaged, and secondly I returned to Cambridge as a medical student, and therefore by definition with no or little money. However I discovered during that first year in Cambridge that if I could organise a party of 12 people for a Murison Small chalet party, I would get a free holiday. This I did, and therefore returned to Switzerland the next Easter to a chalet at Saas Fe. Most of the people in the party I knew, and the others were made up of people who had answered an advertisement in 'The Times'. And so after warming up on the Saturday I went to join Class V. There was a very brief selection test which somehow I passed. My new instructor was an interesting man who was the local forester, and as we got to know him, he was clearly more of a mountaineer than a ski instructor. In my class were two people with whom I remained in contact. One was the manager of the Hong

Kong and Shanghai Bank in London. When I was back in London he invited me to a lunch at a special Chinese restaurant in London. I met him in his office and he asked me if I would mind if one of his customers joined us. As he was paying, I obviously had no problems, and in fact I met a very unusual young lady, Anna Minton-Beddoes. She had set up orphanages in South Africa – from which she was deported for anti-apartheid reasons, and then another in Hong Kong from which she had just returned. I went out with her for some weeks, and then she departed to Saudi Arabia to set up another orphanage. The other person I met was John Flynn. We skied together for several years afterwards, and as an architect he helped me with several of my building works. We are still in touch. The skiing that I particularly mention was with our instructor who leant us sets of skins to attach to our skis. We then walked uphill from the top of the ski lift for about two hours, turned round and skied downhill in deep snow for about ten minutes to where we started. Ski mountaineering rapidly disappeared off my list of things to do in the future, but am still sorry that I did not do the Haute Route ski tour – I think.

The next year I organised a group to ski in Verbier, again in a Murison Small chalet. The two chalet girls were Liz and Sarah. Sarah Yates was a nurse having a ski season away. John Flynn went out with her for some time and she then disappeared to work in Cape Town. I arranged to meet her there where she was working as the theatre sister to Christiaan Barnard. She organised me to go into the theatre to see him operate – not that time doing a heart transplant. Liz was a medical secretary who worked for Mr Frank Ellis, a renowned vascular and transplant surgeon at Guy's Hospital in London. Liz organised me to meet him and to watch him operate. This I did, and on the first occasion when he finished the operation he told me to go to the next door theatre where his registrar was doing a mastectomy. This caused me the most frightening episode in my medical career up to then, and perhaps for the whole of my career. There had been two changing rooms – one for senior surgeons and one for more junior surgeons and medical students. They had different hats allocated to each, and as I had been with Mr Ellis, I had a senior hat on. When I walked into the registrar's theatre, the anaesthetist took one look at me, and said,

"Look after the patient I am having a cup of tea," and walked out. The registrar smiled and said if there was a problem he would tell me what to do. After half an hour of my panic the anaesthetist returned, and I told him that I was a pre-clinical medical student. He smiled and said,

"Well the patient is OK."

The next time I visited Mr Ellis a couple of weeks later, I again went to see his registrar operating, and as I walked in the anaesthetist looked at me and said,

"Oh it's you again – so I am off for my cup of tea."

The skiing in Verbier was excellent, and I particularly remember Mont Géle. There were two very black (for experts only) deep snow runs down from the top with the warning that rescue was by helicopter only. On only my third skiing trip I did the slightly easier of the two. My other memory of that trip was meeting a young lady, Diana Samways, at the Ski Club of Great Britain (SCGB) party. We got on well and she suggested that we ski together the next day. What Diana had not told me was that she was an excellent skier and although a GP, skied for six months each year. She was the first lady, and also the first English person, to qualify for the Swiss Ski Patrol. I had an excellent lesson and we remain in touch.

The next year the trip was to Kitzbuhel at Christmas rather than Easter. I have a memory of watching a ski procession carrying torches coming down the slope to the village one night. What I do not remember was knocking myself out – and several hours of my life disappeared. I am told I skied over a precipice in fog. Luckily there were doctors on the trip who looked after me. With the Ski Club we did go down the track of the famous Hahnenkamm race which is acknowledged as the most difficult race of all – but we were not racing. My other memory there was a ski lift that got stuck half way up the mountain. The person sharing the chair with me was Toni Sailer, a previous multiple World champion who was warming up for the season to come. We had a long conversation, but unfortunately he did not offer to give me a lesson.

The penultimate group tour that I organised was to Zermatt which was a marvellous return for me – now considerably more experienced and able to enjoy all of the relatively easy black runs. The SCGB had a series of awards to measure one's skills. One of these was a timed downhill race. Both John Flynn and I did our silver level races and other parts of the test. The Ski Club rep made a timing mistake on my downhill run, and I had to repeat it. My second time broke the record for that run.

Having qualified for the silver award of the Ski Club in 1970 I was selected to join the Representative's Course which was to occur in Davos in December 1971. It turned out to be the highlight of my skiing, both at the time and in the future. There were 16 students, with four instructors, three of whom had skied for Britain in the Olympics of various years. Also with us was the President of the Ski Club of Great Britain, Jimmy Riddle, again an ex-Olympian. We travelled out by train, itself an interesting experience and stayed in a very smart hotel – far smarter than anywhere before or since when skiing. Skiing was early morning until dusk, we then had a meal which was followed by lectures. On one interesting day we also visited the Swiss state avalanche research laboratory. With extreme luck at the beginning of December, the snow was absolutely ideal; with fresh snow falling during several nights. The course itself included a variety of skiing including downhill racing, slalom and a large amount of off piste skiing. The instructors were brilliant, and certainly by the end of each day most of us were too exhausted to do anything but go to sleep. The skiing included, where it was possible, a chance for us to advance to the gold level of the Ski Club. The slalom skiing, which I had not done, was a real challenge. Part of the course was learning to set courses for skiers of different levels of ability, which with some elementary trigonometry is not difficult. The off piste skiing was difficult because of the great depth of the new snow that had fallen and continued to fall. To pass the deep snow test for the gold award one had to descend a certain height with only three falls. Unfortunately I (and nearly all of us) failed to do this. The so-called crash and dash, i.e. the downhill race, was more successful and I passed this relatively easily. The third part of the gold award was, and is, varied snow. This means leading a class down the best route through a variety of snow, ideally some deep snow, some ice, and any other variety of snow that occurs. Unfortunately, because of the continual falling of snow, this part of the award was not possible and none of us therefore added it to their record. The evening lectures included first aid, and one of our instructors was Neil Orr, a consultant surgeon from Colchester. He in fact was the only instructor who was not an ex-Olympian, but for his National Service had spent 18 months in the Antarctic as a medical officer with the research teams that were working there. He was a superb skier, particularly off piste. Another memory I have of that week was watching our 70 year old President Jimmy ski down an almost vertical slope. His head would go down almost without moving, and the rest of his body would waggle underneath in total control. Then on the last day we had an incredible ski as a group from the top of Davos to Klosters, a distance of about 12 miles with no stopping. At the end of the course I was told that I had qualified both as a future rep and also a judge for slalom skiing. Unfortunately I have never used either as both a marriage and work got in the way.

Vivian and I became engaged two weeks after returning from the course. I had already organised a chalet with ten other people for the next Easter in Crans-Montana, and this became our first honeymoon. Somewhat unusual to spend it with ten friends, but at least they allowed us the only double bed in the chalet. Vivian had only had one previous skiing holiday and therefore went off to a class whilst I skied with my friends. Because the weather was too warm the skiing was relatively poor. I had my binoculars with me, and for the first time Vivian discovered my passion for bird-watching.

Vivian and I then skied almost every year apart from our year in Australia until Covid came along. In the next few years our skiing holidays were with friends and then when our daughters were old enough they were inseparable from the snow and are now extremely competent skiers. We have skied in Austria at St Anton, France in Chamonix and Tignes, Switzerland in Val-d'Isere, Verbier and Ovrannaz, and also tried some more unusual resorts of Pamparovo in Bulgaria, Ortisei in Italy, Soldeu in Andorra and even Whistler in Canada. These holidays produced some memorable occasions. In Chamonix we nearly lost the children. We had arranged to meet them after their ski class which somehow finished up at a different destination to that arranged. In Ovrannaz we used the chalet Elephant Blanc which belonged to Donald Wyzenbeck, an artist friend of Vivian's brother John, and this time we nearly lost Johns' young children. I had taken them down the hill in our car in a vicious snowstorm and returned rapidly before being stuck out. When I returned it became apparent that we had missed the fact that the clocks had gone forward at the end of winter, and the train they were due to catch, and for which they had tickets, had already left an hour earlier. Very luckily a helpful local gentleman managed to sort out their return journey. In Andorra where we joined the Royal Navy Ski Club, the skiing was very basic, but luckily there was a man in the chalet who liked off-piste skiing and we immediately linked up. On one occasion a car in the car park below our chalet was intentionally damaged. The police arrived and immediately picked on the one younger person in our party as the culprit – perhaps because he was a long haired undergraduate. They confiscated his passport and were not going to return it until the cost of the damage was paid. He was completely innocent as he had been with us all the time, but to save him going to prison we had a collection and paid the money. Surprise, surprise we have not been to Andorra since. In Ortisei a lift was out of action which meant that between lifts there was a long somewhat uphill walk. When asked when the lift was to be repaired, a blank look, and then the information that it might be before next year. In Bulgaria we stayed in a very Russian looking hotel with an enormous menu in three languages. English was not one, but luckily Vivian had fluent German. She translated for me and we made our choices.

"Not today," was the response. So we chose again.

"Not today." It eventually turned out that there was no choice and one item each day of each course was available. At least very edible. My other memory was again bird watching and seeing for the first and only time a black woodpecker.

Many years later when we were living in Whitchurch in Buckinghamshire we were invited by Sir Edward and Lady Tomkins to join them in their chalet in Meribel. They said that they would very much wish to have two doctors in the party. It turned out that the other people in the party were the Duke of Kent, James Elles MEP and Peter and Leonie Thorogood. Edward Tomkins was a very interesting man. Meribel was created and developed by Col Peter Lindsay and the Count de la Valdenne in the 1930s, and Edward, whose mother was French, became involved as a director and very early chalet owner. He had been a very expert skier himself but very tragically when we knew him he was nearly eighty years old and was losing his sense of balance, and was unable to ski. The rest of the party which included the Duke, were all experts. Vivian was very much the least expert – closely followed by me. The evenings with games including Trivial Pursuits were a real challenge – and the Duke, Vivian and I were then the more expert. This party was repeated for the next two years. On one occasion the Duke and Duchess of Bedford were coming as dinner guests. Unfortunately the Duchess, a somewhat large lady, slipped on her way up the drive. Peter went to help her, and put one arm round each of her sides, at which point she turned around, looked at him and said,

"I do not think that we have been introduced." Peter, considerably embarrassed, was wondering what to do next when she started laughing. A marvellous and very amusing evening followed. The Bedfords really should have been comedians.

In 2000, apart from one visit to Whistler, skiing for us moved to Verbier. On our retirement from the NHS Vivian and I decided to buy a ski chalet/apartment somewhere. France with its peculiar inheritance laws was less than ideal, and hence we chose Switzerland. With the two children when they were young we had rented a chalet in Verbier, and that was our first choice. We had some money from our retirement package, and also from the sale of the Old House. We had some problems with the local bank proving that the money was not laundered,

SCHOLARSHIP BOY TO ENGINEER, PLASTIC SURGEON AND SPORTSMAN

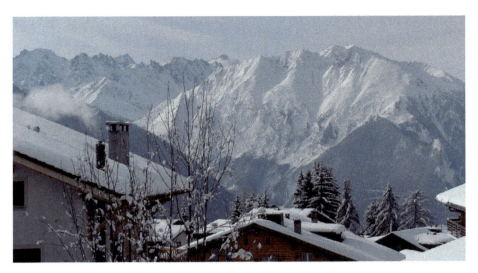

20.1 Verbier, the view from our ski chalet.

and an interesting experience when we went to the solicitors to pay for the apartment. We were told that if we took 10% of the money in a brown envelope it would be sold to us for a cheaper price. And we had always thought that the country was honest. After purchase we immediately gave the apartment to our daughters. Now long past the seven years it is fully theirs (Photo 20.1).

We have had some marvellous holidays there, and especially as the lift ticket is free when one is over 75, and also covers several surrounding smaller resorts so that one never needs to be bored. As well as skiing there is snowboarding, skating, climbing which includes an indoor wall, and also paragliding. The last is not something that I had considered but one Christmas my daughters, with no warning, gave me my Christmas present which was a session. I had no option, and therefore set off in tandem with my skis on with the instructor and we landed by the bottom of the main lift in the valley some ten minutes later. When Tasha married Jumbo he already had a chalet in Verbier and they have since had another larger one built. That one won the prize for the architect for the best new chalet in the Alps that year.

I was determined to ski when I was eighty year old, and just managed it before Covid in effect closed the Alps for people from the United Kingdom.

A marvellous sport, and an excellent way of holidaying with family and friends. Our daughter Tasha did two seasons working in Verbier, and both our daughters met their husbands skiing.

I had the serious head injury but apart from some sore muscles no other injuries. Vivian was less lucky and after one bad fall when her skies did not come off, she fractured a knee and an ankle. But she returned to skiing the next year.

TWENTY-ONE

SAILING

And now for something completely different. Sailing. Having had to swim at school and in the scouts, and succeeded at a fair level, having failed as a scuba diver and again with a minor interest in canoeing and kayaking, sailing became my major sport – in the scouts, at university, and for many years afterwards until 1971. Even in the 70s to compete at a high level one had to sail every weekend and several weeks a year in the championships. Work in particular and also married life then reduced my serious sailing. I sailed only three times until I returned to sailing in 1997. One of the reasons for buying an apartment and then moving to the Isle of Wight was the sailing. Back to sailing I went, and Vivian started almost as a complete novice. At the age of 83 I am still teaching people to sail but no longer competing in races.

Sailing boats are categorised in several ways.

They can have one hull or several hulls (a catamaran with two, or a trimaran with three).

They can have a fixed keel or keels (a yacht) or a centreboard or centreplate (a dinghy).

All boats can be used for cruising or racing. Boats used for racing are divided up into classes which have fixed rules for size, sail area, weight etc. In different dinghy classes all boats may either be identical, or built within close limits. Alternatively all yachts and dinghy classes are given an international handicap so that racing can take place between boats or classes.

As did so many other things in my life sailing started for me in the scouts. I joined the 36th Epping Forest South group at the age of eight in 1946. Sailing started with a trip to Holland in 1951 when we sailed in small sailing cruising yachts for two weeks. This was repeated the next year, and by that time I was able to rig and sail a boat. The group had two small wooden dinghies which were sailed at Maylandsea Bay Yacht Club on the River Blackwater in Essex. In about 1955 Graham Taylor, a friend in my class at Bancroft's School, had his own Cadet class racing dinghy which he sailed on lagoons at Broxbourne Sailing Club on the River Lea in Essex. Sailing with Graham was my introduction to sailing a racing dinghy, and the Cadet was the ideal boat. They were designed by Jack Holt in 1947 for two children up to the age of seventeen. They were different to sail than the boats that I had previously sailed in that the helm and the crew sat on the deck to keep the boat upright, and they also had spinnakers. The class grew rapidly around the world and is still raced, particularly overseas.

After returning from the expedition to Arctic Finland I went to Leeds University (Chapter 1) and joined the University Sailing Club for the princely sum of 5/- (25p) a year. John Stork, who had recently come out of the Royal Navy having finished his National Service, had founded the club the previous year with Stuart King-Cox and David Daish amongst others. In the first years the dinghies were privately owned and a mixture of classes. Sailing was on Roundhay Lake on one afternoon a week and at the weekend. In my first year the University bought two Firefly dinghies for the club. Numbers 506 and 693. The Firefly was designed by Uffa Fox in 1946 for two people, but was surprisingly selected as the single-handed boat for the 1948 Olympics in Torbay, and which was won by the famous Danish sailor Paul Elvstrom. The original boats were carvel built (where the planks do not overlap) of cold moulded wood. Nearly all universities in the UK adopted them as the team boat.

The other boats that we had at Roundhay in 1957 were the National 12s of John Stork and of Mike Purton, a Firefly, and an International 14' belonging to David Milns. This was a very old boat named 'Afterthought' number K371. The amazing thing about this boat was that, especially in light winds, it was about twice as fast as the 12" boats on Roundhay Lake. What would be a total surprise to any sailor now were the clothes that we then wore. Wet-suits may have been invented but had not spread to sailors, and as the waterproofs were fairly heavy and used for sea cruising and long distance racing, were not suitable for dinghy sailing. Therefore shorts were normally worn, and possibly a light windcheater – even when it was snowing.

SCHOLARSHIP BOY TO ENGINEER, PLASTIC SURGEON AND SPORTSMAN

Most of the sailing in that first year was teaching the new recruits to sail, and this often led to some interesting capsizes. One that I well remember was a young lass on her first sail who panicked somewhat when the boat capsized. It turned out that she could not swim, but was luckily wearing a lifejacket. To help her Alan Birch put out a hand when sailing past, but instead of him pulling her into his boat, she pulled him into the water. His boat, with another complete beginner, then sailed serenely across the lake without capsizing until it ran aground. The rule nowadays is that even in a complete calm, lifejackets must be worn in all Royal Yachting Association clubs. Perhaps Health and Safety can sometimes go too far.

As the years progressed people graduated or moved on, and new undergraduates joined. It was noticeable that a greater percentage of new undergraduates had had previous sailing experience. Each year at the beginning of the autumn term the new students had to be assessed to determine their ability, and to possibly select them for a team. I well remember one young lad who was extremely keen to impress. He was crewing for me when a sudden gust came. He shot out to keep the boat upright but missed the toe straps and did a very elegant back dive into the lake, and without even splashing me. He actually did turn out to a be very good sailor.

Over the next four years whilst I was at Leeds the club went from strength to strength. We acquired six Firefly dinghies through the sports fund of the Students' Union, and also somewhere to keep them and to upkeep them by revarnishing etc. We found that a more effective way of doing the revarnishing was to lend a boat to a member to be used in the national championships during the summer vacation, providing that they scraped and revarnished it. I did this during two summer vacations.

Sailing on the lake in the autumn and winter terms was still the main experience, and in the summer we also sailed at Burwain Sailing Club on the top of the Pennines. This gave good competition and was an excellent day out at weekends. The other thing that we did as a club in my last two years was to hire cruising boats on the Norfolk Broads. A very different experience for most of us. There were several stories that could be told, but one I remember was when we returned to the boatyard at the end of the week all the boats were examined for damage. Amazingly the yard manager then gave us some money back with the comment that there had been no damage at all, and that that was unique in his experience.

Team racing normally has six people, most commonly three helms and three crew, although the helms and crews can change roles for each race. Team racing was an important part of all university sailing, and Leeds rapidly joined in. A racing team was started to compete against other universities and local clubs, and because of its new foundation there was a shortage of crews to go with the few experienced helmsmen. I therefore rapidly walked into the team. Because of the previous experience of our helms the team was very successful from the start. Our first team-racing that first year was away matches only with other universities or clubs because to hold home matches we would need six boats of the same class. In my second year, by which time I was established as a crew and as an occasional helmsman, we had our six boats and were competing in Leeds, as far north as Tyneside, and as far south as London as well as at Oxford and Cambridge – and still winning more than 50% of the matches. Our team changed over the years Having started with John Stork and Stuart King Cox it included myself, David Milns, Peter Schroeder, Cherry James, John Franklin, Pat Langridge and in my last year, Mike Carroll and Mike Cobb – two dental students. Cherry was also a dental student with whom I remained in touch and who tragically died in her late thirties from a brain tumour. I have remained in touch with both Johns, David, and Peter.

The other thing that became obvious was that it was an excellent way of meeting young ladies.

In 1959 we competed in the Association of Northern University Sailing Clubs (ANUSC) championship and won it. The next year the ANUSC championship was in Dublin. We also competed in the British Universities Sailing Association (BUSA) championships which were held on The Welsh Harp reservoir in north London – but somewhat less successfully. Within the LUSC I was awarded my half colours in my third year, and full colours in my final year. And then to my amazement in that final year I was selected for the British Universities team to sail against the French Universities. Even more amazing was that Graham Taylor from my form at school, who was captaining London University at the time, was also selected. What are the chances of that? The competition occurred in Vaurien dinghies on a branch of the Seine (I believe the Marne) a few miles east of Paris. The boat had been designed and was a basic early chine design for two people which was very popular in France. Clearly it also suited British sailors as we won very easily. The day ended with a dinner on a marvellous barge on the Seine, and afterwards on the way back to our hotel, and with some alcohol in us both, I challenged Richard Keith – another member of the team – to a race up the 222 steps leading to the Sacre-Coeur Cathedral. Totally exhausted I won the race by two steps. I also remember Colin, Richard's brother, climbing up a tree to pick some mistletoe to show some young French lasses that it had a very important use.

As well as the sailing I became involved in positions within the clubs. In LUSC I was secretary, then vice-commodore and finally commodore. It was a very sociable club and I am still in contact with several of the members, and remained in contact with some of the lady members until their deaths in the last few years. Of those I particularly remember Roz Nixon and Liz Pirie. Another girlfriend and my crew for many matches was Anne Everett. On one occasion the team were sailing against London, and some of the team were staying in our house. This included Anne. My Aunt Dot was visiting and thought that Anne was my girlfriend – which was somewhat true. Anne was incredibly innocent and did not realise that Aunt Dot was trying to find out about her. Certainly Aunt Dot was extremely impressed when Anne told her that she lived in a Georgian mansion with twenty bedrooms. My aunt however never discovered that her father was the owner and headmaster of a preparatory school in Wiltshire! Within ANUSC I became secretary, and within BUSA was assistant secretary.

It must be obvious that I was stricken with the sport, and that I was reasonably competent. In the 1930s the only class of dinghy regularly raced was the International 14 foot dinghy. These were expensive and to provide a cheaper option the Royal Yachting Association produced the rules for a 12 foot maximum length boat with two sails up to a defined maximum area. It was decided that it would be a restricted class and would therefore develop with time. The first boats were built in 1936 and were designed by a variety of people. After the Second World War Ian Proctor became the most prolific designer for several years. I committed to sailing even more seriously by requesting only money for my 21st birthday, and with the presents and a little of my own, I built a National 12' dinghy. Built is not quite the correct word. I bought the shell of a Proctor Mk 8 design from Wyche and Coppock, and put on the decks, the transom, the buoyancy and all the fixtures and rigging. This was all done in the sitting room of our bungalow as we no longer had paying guests once the mortgage had been paid off, and my mother allowed me so to use it. Luckily there were double doors onto the lawn, and the dinghy just fitted through when it was finished. I called her Totora, the Latin name for the reed (probably bulrush) used on Lake Titicaca for building boats, and popularized by the Danish author Thor Heyerdahl. He used a reed boat to sail from Peru to Easter Island. The boat was successfully measured and received the number

1885 within the class. I then needed somewhere to sail it. I considered Maylandsea Bay Yacht Club where I had sailed as a scout, but they did not have a National 12 fleet. I therefore looked at and joined the Thames Estuary Yacht Club. This was based at Westcliff on Sea, in fact on the Thames Estuary, a journey by road from home of about 35 miles. They had an active National 12 class with about 20 boats and I sailed Totora whenever I was at home for a weekend, and I also took her to two Burton weeks, the national championships of National 12' class dinghies (Photo 21.1).

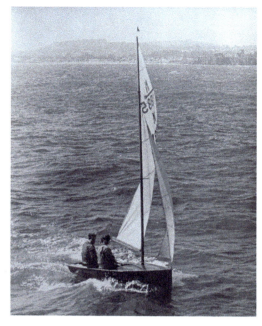

21.1 My National 12' dinghy at Torquay with Anne Cox crewing me.

In September 1961 I went to Cambridge and immediately joined the Cambridge University Cruising Club which had been founded in 1893. Originally developed for cruising during vacations, but over the years had also taken up dinghy sailing and racing. On arrival I was told that I was to be the new secretary in succession to Dr Roger Needham (later Sir Roger) who had held the post for many years and saw an obvious opportunity to resign. I do not remember being asked whether I was interested, but I was instantly appointed.

In 1961 the dinghy sailing was on the River Cam at St Ives. This was a narrow river with trees and buildings on one side, and fishermen on the other side. It was difficult sailing because of the multitudinous wind shifts and also trying to avoid the fishermen. I well remember one day when there was a fishing competition occurring and the fishermen were becoming extremely frustrated at having to withdraw their floats every time a boat passed. However one fisherman discovered that every time he reeled in there was a fish on the end of his line, and after he had won the competition he actually thanked us. The sailing was on the river for the whole of my first year in Cambridge. We had a boatyard there run by delightful old man with a wealth of stories. The next year after negotiation we moved to the gravel pits in St Ives. Certainly the sailing was easier, which was sometimes a disadvantage as visiting teams did not need the specialist knowledge that we had used when on the river.

Until that year the club had used Firefly dinghies on the river and the gravel pit, but we also owned a 15 foot Swordfish dinghy (No. 1) which was kept at the Royal Harwich Yacht Club on the Orwell River for occasional use in the summer. The Swordfish had been the two man Olympic dinghy for the 1948 Games in Torquay and was a lengthened Firefly.

I do not remember how the club was persuaded to invest in the new Alpha dinghy, which they did along with the Royal Navy and the Oxford University Yacht Club as well as a few private owners. This was a 12 foot fibreglass boat based on the Proctor Mark VIII National 12 foot dinghy. The advantages were said to be much easier maintenance, which was true, and as the construction was two layers of fibreglass with foam between them, no matter how damaged it was it would be unsinkable. These advantages sounded excellent, but very rapidly the two layers of fibreglass separated and the gap filled with water, making the boat considerably heavier. As they became heavier they became more difficult to sail, particularly in a strong wind. When it was really blowing the only way of sailing them off wind was for the helmsman to sit on the transom, and for the crew to sit on their lap. We had one very interesting race against the Thorpe Bay Yacht Club whose team consisted of Keith Musto, an Olympic silver medallist, Kit Hobday, the World Hornet dinghy champion, and the third sailor was I believe Peter Bateman, a winner of the Endeavour trophy. That trophy was presented to the winner each year of a competition between the champions of all the various dinghy classes. It was blowing a good hoolie and needless to say we did not tell the opposition about the problems. In the four races two of their team capsised in each race, and Keith was the only one of their team that finished a race upright. Needless to say we won easily. The second half of this story was the return match at Thorpe Bay on the River Thames estuary which was normally held in the very basic GP 14 dinghies. When we arrived they announced that there would be a change and that year it would be held in Hornet dinghies. These were almost unique in that the crew was able to sit or lie on a sliding wooden seat which gave them a much better purchase to keep the boat upright, later to be replaced by the trapeze. Kit was the international Hornet champion, and only one of our team had ever used a sliding seat. Needless to say revenge from their disastrous match against us was achieved – but the result was considerably closer.

Another race that I remember was against a team from, I think, Reading University. They arrived by train at Cambridge and the six of us in our team all had interesting open cars. We collected one member each and then drove to the gravel pit. The car park there was gravel, and we had all practised turns and backwards parking many times. When we did this with our unsuspecting passengers, they were sufficiently frightened that they were no competition at all in the sailing match.

In my four years at Cambridge we had some excellent sailors in the team which included the successive captains John Thompson, Peter Bainbridge and Richard Hermon-Taylor. I believe that we lost very few matches indeed. Our away matches were sometimes made more interesting as Chris Cockcroft in our team would borrow the Bentley of his father, Sir John Cockcroft, the Nobel prize winner, to take half the team to the match. We travelled in style. We also entered the British Universities Championships at the Welsh Harp in London and one year we were the runners-up. The most important match of every year was against our old rivals at Oxford. It is a great regret that I was not able to be in this team as I had already had four years of university sailing before Cambridge, and the rules therefore excluded me. Roy Williams, who was a brilliant sailor, had come from Nottingham University and because he had only been there for three years did win his half blue in his first year at Cambridge. Within my college Graham Self, who came from The Broads, sailed on occasions for the university. He joined us for annual cruising weeks at Easter with the club (Photo 21.2).

The Wilson team trophy which is regarded as the principal sailing team event in the world occurs each year at the West Kirby Sailing Club on the Wirral Peninsula in Lancashire. It occurs during exam time

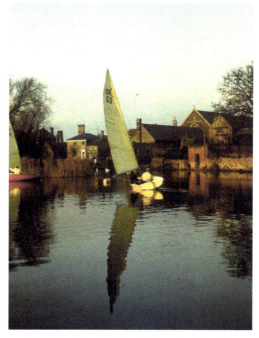

21.2 The Cambridge University Cruising Club on the Norfolk Broads in 1963. A very different form of sailing.

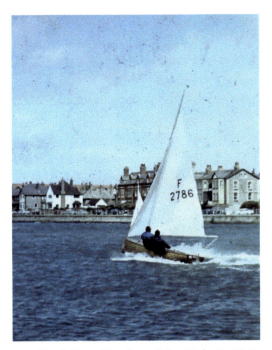

at universities and the team representing Cambridge therefore consisted of graduates studying for higher degrees. I captained this team twice. The first time we were beaten in the semi-final, and the second time in a howling gale we lost to the Oxford and Cambridge Sailing Society in the first round, but were the only team to beat them in one race on their way to success as winners (Photo 21.3).

21.3 The Wilson Trophy at West Kirby in 1963. A reefed Firefly dinghy in very strong winds.

As well as being very successful on the water it was an incredibly friendly club with premises at 5 Falcon Yard in the centre of Cambridge, and I am still in contact with several members. Our club room was on the second floor and was overseen by the redoubtable Mrs Hobbs who ran the bar and served coffee. On the wall was a painting by Sir Peter Scott that he had given to the club when he had been a member as an undergraduate. He went on to win a bronze medal for sailing in the 1936 Olympics. The floor above us was occupied by the famous Footlights Club who would try out their new acts at our 'smokers' (what a dreadful thought that is now). If we approved of them, they would then perform the act at various theatres around the country. One of their famous members was John Cleese and my memory of him was that he gatecrashed with a young lady one of our 'smokers', and left very rapidly when he realised that it was a bachelor event. As he left I poured a large glass of water over his head. It had seemed a good idea at the time. Another memory from there was giving one of our team, Roger Palmer, a quick tutorial in chemistry as he was going into his examination. He thanked me profusely afterwards as the subject, about which he had known very little, was one of the questions. The club in the 1960s and 70s was all male, but sailing was an excellent way of meeting lady undergraduates who were welcome in the club room, and in particular I met a girlfriend, Jane Caroe, through sailing. One other marvellous memory was an annual dinner where the guest was the famous sailor, Uffa Fox. With a generous amount of alcohol in him he stood up and thanked our captain and Vice-Commodore Richard Hormone Taylor for the invitation. It should have been Hermon-Taylor, and whether it was a deliberate mistake we will never know. It was however a very appropriate change of name and we used his new name from then on.

Some years later I captained a Sea View Yacht Club team who were due to sail against Cambridge at their new home on Grafham Water. When we arrived it was blowing a force eight gale. The Grafham committee obviously thought nobody would be so stupid as to sail in the conditions and had not put up a no sailing flag. Peter Hunter, a very well-known dinghy crew and I, having driven a hundred and twenty miles to get to Grafham were not to be frustrated and launched a dinghy. We had a marvellous sail in the gale which was still rising. It was eventually measured as gusting a force 10. Various other people in both teams thought that if we could do it so could they, but nobody lasted more than about 30 seconds before capsizing. The club then put up the no sailing flag.

In 1962 whilst I was secretary at Cambridge I received a letter from the Sea View Yacht Club advertising a post as assistant secretary of that club for the month of August. The letter said that the pay was five pounds a week, there was free board and lodging and as much sailing as one could fit in. I forgot to put it on our notice board and applied for the post. Looking back that letter made an enormous difference to my future life. Firstly it revolutionised my sailing possibilities and also my social life as it led to a flat mate and many friends in London, and later in life to moving to the Isle of Wight where we have now lived for the past twenty years.

Sea View Yacht Club was founded in 1893, which by chance was the same year as the Cambridge University Cruising Club. It is situated on the north east coast of the Isle of Wight. In the 1960s it was very selective as to its membership, as somebody recently put it, trade was not electable, and also nobody under the age of 12 was allowed into the club. The children with their nannies used to sit on the sea wall outside the club waiting for their parents. Another anomaly of the club for that time was that the yachts were owned by the club. They were extremely well used as the club rented them out to the Services or to other organisations, for instance the Law Society, during weekdays from Easter until the end of July. Members could rent them for evening races or at weekends and then had full use of the yachts during August. The thirteen yachts are known as Seaview Mermaids and were designed in 1907, are 30 feet long and have a spinnaker. They are normally sailed by three people, but can be easily managed by two. The original boats were built from wood with carvel construction. When I was there in 1962 the wooden boats had just been replaced with glassfibre boats which are still used today.

The club also had a class of clinker built small dinghies which were individually owned. These boats are 12 foot long and can be sailed by either one or two people, including cadets. They are normally kept on moorings and taken out for storage during the winter. A total of just over 200 have been built since they were designed in 1931. The majority of these had been built by the local boat builder Warren and Sons whose yard touches on to the clubhouse. If a severe northeast gale is forecast they are taken out of the water and stored on the local road. This happened once during my stay in 1962 when a selection of people came to help us move them all to safety.

In 1962 I had trailed my National 12" foot dinghy from home and having taken my car across on the small car ferry then returned to the Portsmouth Sailing Club who had very kindly allowed me to leave my trailer there for the month. I then sailed the boat single-handed across the Solent. My job for the month was to assist the secretary Lt-Col Mossy McLeod-Carey. This was partly in the office, collecting the subs from the members, and also helping Mr Daish the boatman in his shed and regularly running the motorboat to take the sailors from the shore to the moored Mermaids. Very soon I was also running the races. A friend of mine Barry Hook told me some time later that the secretary had some trouble keeping me busy. He would give me work for two days and half a day later I would go back to the office asking for further work. Clearly it was not what he was used to. The accommodation was in a small room in which there were four bunks for males only. The food was served in the clubhouse but very rapidly I was receiving invitations to dine with members of the club, and particularly when they had daughters. I am not sure if this was at the suggestion of the daughters or whether the mothers thought that a postgraduate Cambridge student might be a suitable husband. There were in fact some very attractive young ladies who included Vicky Asprey, Clare Francis, Eve Bonham and Claire Jensen (and somehow I have not forgotten their names). I discovered afterwards that the Cambridge undergraduate who had done the job the year before had become engaged and later married one of the young ladies of the club.

Having settled in I managed to do some sailing and particularly crewing for members in the Mermaids, and occasionally for the younger cadets in the dinghies. This included the famous round the world racer and later author Clare Francis, and I like to think that I contributed to her ability to race. There was no handicap class suitable for racing with my National 12', and over the next few weeks with Dr John Almond, who owned a Merlin Rocket, and Arthur Birchenough, who owned a Wayfarer dinghy, we started a small handicap class. We were soon joined by Barry Hook with his Fireball dinghy and later by several other sailors. The handicap class is still running today.

It was excellent month which I very much enjoyed. At the end I dropped hints that I would like to become a member of the club and was told to find a suitable proposer and seconder. By this stage I had become friendly with several of the more senior members and Sir Edward Blount proposed me and Lt Col Longland seconded me. I am pleased to say that with those people I was elected a member without any problem. Perhaps I was not trade after all, or they had not found out about it.

The next year the job was done by Richard Prest who was already a member of the club, and was later to become Commodore. That summer I taught sailing for the Youth Hostel Association. I had obviously enjoyed myself so much at Seaview that I returned in the summer of 1964. At that time I was just about to start my university lectureship in London. Mossy had retired as secretary, and there was a very newly retired RAF officer. It turned out that part of my job was to teach him his job. The sailing was still the same, the handicap class was thriving and it had been joined by an Alpha dinghy of the same class that was causing the chaos in Cambridge. This was owned and sailed by the Surridge sisters. One very positive thing that came out of my month in Seaview was that I was introduced by Barry Hook to an old college friend of his, Peter Burgess, who by chance was looking for a flatmate to join him and a colleague in London. I immediately signed up.

In the 1960s there were strange relations between some of the clubs in the island, and particularly between the Bembridge Sailing club and Sea View Yacht Club. It was said that Bembridge had the titles and Seaview had the money – by no means strictly true. During the month of August in 1964 I went out on occasions with a Bembridge girl, Antonia Bennet, and was nearly thrown out of the Sea View Yacht Club. Antonia, or Toni as she was normally known, was a very unusual girl. When she went to Oxford the following year she was a major leader of the student unrest strikes and eventually married

Red Robbo who was the British Leyland steward who organised the major strike in the factory in Oxford. By this time I had lost contact with Toni, and I am sure that her father, Sir Reginald Bennet, who was a Conservative member of Parliament, would have been upset by his daughter's behaviour. Another chance story about Bembridge occurred many years later when I was operating in a Milton Keynes Hospital and was talking to the theatre sister who was assisting me. During the conversation she mentioned that she had sailed at Bembridge when she was a young girl.

"You must have a title," was my instant comment, at which point she blushed somewhat and said,

"Well actually I do, but nobody knows about it."

We laughed a little and I kept her secret.

I also did occasional sailing with the scouts during some university vacations. For this I had to take a scout association test which I did on the River Blackwater in a Firefly. This was nearly a disaster as the person examining me was very obviously unused to small racing dinghies. He arrived with his sea scout hat on and sat in the middle of the boat. On the first tack the boom knocked his hat off and I managed to catch it before it went into the water, and he did not move again. He passed me very rapidly. But ridiculously that scout licence only covered the water on which it was taken, and I therefore had to pass another test on Lake Windermere so that I could sail with the 40th N W Leeds Rover Scouts from the university. This I did on a few occasions and rapidly learnt that Windermere, where the wind comes from all directions and in variable force, is not easy sailing. And finally in my last summer vacation I taught sailing for the Youth Hostels Association at their Maldon sailing centre on the River Blackwater in Essex. The warden there was Dougie Lamb and the boats that they used were West Country Redwings – not to be confused with the Bembridge Redwings. The National Redwing as it came to be known is a carvel built wooden dinghy 14' long, and was designed by Uffa Fox in the late 1930s to withstand the seas and winds off the Cornish coast. It was an excellent boat to teach young and complete beginners. One memory I have of that visit was sailing into the harbour at Bradwell-on-Sea where the nuclear reactor was later built. Dougie had told me how to get into the harbour which was only possible at high tide in many boats, and that the deeper water was on the far east side of the 100 yard wide channel. As I sailed in a larger cruising boat followed me, and when we had moored he thanked me – as an expert – for showing him the channel. He said that he had been trying to get in for the past two hours and had run aground on the very soft Blackwater mud several times. He looked a little shocked when I told him that it was my first entry to the harbour. Luckily Dougie had told me to keep a marker pole in line with the church steeple as the two necessary guide marks.

As soon as I had moved into the flat in Earls Court and started lecturing I was looking for somewhere to sail in the winter and joined the London Corinthian Sailing Club which was based in Hammersmith in an extremely attractive old building. The club sailed on the River Thames. This was an interesting experience in itself as the river was known to be extremely unhygienic to the degree that not long previously there had been a recommendation that anyone who capsized should spend a day in hospital being cleaned out. I will say that I never came across anybody who had done this. There were several well known members including two that were regularly seen acting on the television. But by far the most interesting was Sir Alan (A P) Herbert the famous author and retired Member of Parliament. It was never confirmed, but the rumour in the club was that he had composed the well known, and somewhat risqué poem 'Eskimo Nell'. The club had no National 12' fleet but an excellent and thriving International 14' fleet. From my university sailing days I had six contacts who sailed International 14's. These were John Stork, Robin Steavenson and David Milns from Leeds days, Neil Spurway from Cambridge, and two sailors that I had sailed against. These were Ken Merron from Oxford and James Vernon from Trinity College Dublin. In 1964 there were no trapezes allowed in the class, and although somewhat light I had crewed with all those helmsman in several races. At the London Corinthian Club I was rapidly taken on as a crew by John Ogle, and I crewed for him for the next three years in London during the winter and on the south coast during the summers. John was a fascinating man who was the financial director of the British American Tobacco (BAC) company, although a total non-smoker. He was a rich man and extremely generous to a new academic who was not very well paid. He fed and watered me very well. As a helmsman in dinghies he was somewhat less successful than the other people I mentioned. The marvellous story about John was that the Chairman of BAT called him into the office one day to congratulate him. John had no idea why he was being congratulated, and was then told by the somewhat puzzled chairman that the reason was that his engagement announcement was in 'The Times' that day. This was a complete surprise to John, and he then worked out that it was February 29, which is the one day in England when every four years the lady may do the proposing. His girlfriend had put the announcement in the paper. He immediately cancelled the arrangement, but did marry her some six months later.

For his summer racing John was a member of the Hayling Island Sailing Club, where a very famous member was the wildlife artist Keith Shackleton, a relative of Sir Ernest Shackleton, the Antarctic explorer, and who sailed a magnificent 10sq.m. canoe. It was a single handed boat with a sliding seat, and definitely one of the most difficult of all dinghies to sail fast. I did borrow it once, but only for a sail and not to race. John and I raced there for that first summer before moving to the Itchenor Sailing Club for the next two summers as the standard of the fleet was much higher, and with several previous winners of the Prince of Wales Cup, which including the Olympic gold medallist Stewart Morris. Stewart had won 12 Prince of Wales cups, far more than anybody else. Among those sailing in the International 14' fleet were my old competitors James Vernon and Keith Merron. We had some interesting sailing but without great success, or in fact any success. I did have one remarkable success when James lent me his 14 and with a young crew who had never put up a spinnaker before I actually beat Stewart Morris in a race.

One other memory was almost being arrested. It was one of the most bizarre stories one could imagine. Sailing in Chichester Harbour with John Ogle in a very strong wind we were dismasted. We were then blown onto the shore which was part of RAF Thorney Island. An RAF policeman arrived and threatened us with arrest if we landed. John somewhat forcibly, but luckily politely enough, told him not to be an idiot as there was absolutely nothing we could do about it, and certainly we did not want to come ashore. Eventually a rescue boat came along and towed us back to Itchenor Sailing Club. On another occasion I had been crewing James Vernon. He suggested on our way back to London that we should drop in to see his parents and have dinner with them. We both had our own cars, and he gave me instructions as to where his parents lived. I followed the instructions and turned left down a small private road. Having driven for about half a mile I came across a magnificent country house. I thought by this stage that I was lost and knocked on the door to ask where the Vernons lived.

"This is their house," said the butler. Considerably taken back I said,

"In that case I have come for dinner."

"Yes sir, would you like to come and change." Needless to say I changed out of my sailing gear into something slightly less scruffy and had a marvellous evening and an excellent dinner with the Vernons. They, for some reason, thought that I was a good influence on James, and I saw them again on occasions when I later shared a flat with him in Chelsea.

In the summer of 1966 I was working at ICI Billingham. There was a well known sailing centre at Tyneside, and I had sailed there against Newcastle University in a freezing winter when I was at Leeds. In summer it looked far more attractive, and I now know not how, but I contacted the best known dinghy sailor in that area, Dr Robin Steavenson, and volunteered my services as his crew. Robin was the only person who had won both the Burton Trophy for National 12s and the Prince of Wales Cup for International 14s. He still had both of his boats and was somewhat keener on sailing the 12. He must have been desperate for a crew as I did manage to persuade him that the 14 would be more fun. We sailed at Tyneside and in a championship on Lake Ullswater in the Lake District. Very enjoyable and I still have a pewter tanker that we won.

One race in which I sailed in my National 12' in 1964 was the first Tideway Race. It started above Hammersmith and went under sixteen bridges, hopefully without hitting one's mast on any of them – which in itself was a challenge. This could only be done on some of them by leaning the boat over considerably. The race was not repeated until 1977 partly because of the worry about the pollution, but it is now an annual event.

My other dinghy sailing during the years at university and in London were in various national championships. Each class holds annual national championships for their members. These are normally moved between the major sailing centres around the country, and are nearly always on the sea and during summer vacations. I took part in several which included Firefly Championships at Weymouth and Gorleston-on-Sea near Yarmouth, in National 12 Championships at Plymouth, Torbay and Scarborough, a Merlin Rocket Championship at Weymouth and Prince of Wales Cups at Scarborough and on the Wash.

Some of these hold special memories. The first that I did was with David Milns at Weymouth. Neither of us had a car at that stage, but we discovered that we could send the boat down by train from Leeds to Weymouth at a remarkably cheap price as the cost was based on weight and not on size. When we collected it we discovered that the varnish had been somewhat damaged and British Railways even paid for the damage to be repaired. In 1958 Fireflies still had cotton sails and when we had pulled the boat on its launching trolley through the streets of Weymouth to the sand there was a Firefly which had just come ashore, and the sails were wet more than half way up.

"Oh have you just capsized?"

"No, "was the reply, "that is just the spray."

Neither David nor I had sailed on the open sea at that stage and we did not quite believe him. Half an hour later we found out that they were indeed telling the truth.

The next Firefly championship in which I sailed was either at Torbay or Plymouth. There was an interesting disaster on I think the first day. It was the first championship in Britain with more than 150 boats, and to mark the occasion a helicopter flew over the fleet to film it. Clearly nobody had realised that the down draught would flatten us all. Not quite 100%, but very nearly.

And the next Firefly championship to which I went was at Gorleston-on-Sea where there is a strong tide that runs along the coast. This was the first meeting that was to try out the recently developed gate start. As the numbers in the fleet had increased the starts had become more chaotic and the new idea was that a selected boat started on port tack, and everybody else could choose when to start crossing on starboard tack astern of the port tack boat. Brian Heron who was the previous year's champion, and by chance had been a member of what was to become my college at Cambridge, was chosen as the port tack boat. The committee got it disastrously wrong in not allowing for the very strong tide, and Brian did not have to tack at all to reach the first mark, and everybody else lost many yards. Later in the week the winds came up. On one day a force 6 wind was forecast to moderate and we went to sea. In fact it increased. When the race was stopped after two legs of the first lap there were three boats left upright with two of them on jib only. Many of the crews had to be rescued from their boats, and it took two days to get all the boats back to the beach. One of the boats that had remained upright on the jib was being sailed by Tessa Wright who had captained Manchester University when I had captained Leeds. She was an Essex girl and we later sailed together on occasions at Maldon on the River Blackwater.

The next interesting championship was the Burton Trophy week of the National 12s. at Plymouth. My flatmate David Brooks was crewing me. David had been involved in a very nasty accident on their farm as a young child and had only half of his right hand. On one day it was blowing hard and the racing was cancelled. I thought that it was an interesting day to go for a sail anyway, but David decided not to come. I was muttering when a young girl said that she would love to crew me. Her name was Ann Cox, and I heard afterwards that as we sailed out of the harbour the Officer of the Day muttered to his wife,

"Who are those idiots going for a sail in this weather?" Knowing perfectly well that it was their daughter she said,

"I don't know dear."

In fact we had an excellent sail and socially the week improved enormously with Ann's local contacts. She later married an orthopaedic hand surgeon colleague of mine.

Either the same year or the next I crewed David Brooks in his Merlin-Rocket 14' dinghy at Weymouth. A pleasant week with one day to be remembered. We were sailing happily along on a gentle plane when the boat took an unexpected course. I turned round to see what David was doing and could see him several yards behind the boat swimming. His missing half of the hand with which he normally coped brilliantly had that day failed him. I turned the boat round and collected him before we carried on.

The other Burton Week that I did was also in Plymouth. At Seaview I had come across an incredible crew, Vicky Asprey. She was extremely able, very fit and without a single nerve in her body. Her mother agreed that she could come to Plymouth as my crew as my mother had agreed to come and to chaperone us. It was an excellent week and I nearly had my best result at any of the championships. I was lying third in a race when the wind failed and the race was cancelled as no one finished within the time allowed.

I crewed in two Prince of Wales weeks for 14' Internationals and the one I remember well was at Scarborough when I crewed for John Stork, the man who had started the Leeds University Sailing Club about ten years earlier. The basic racing rule is that a boat on starboard tack has right of way over a boat on port tack. My memory of that race is that we were on port tack and neither of us had seen a boat approaching on starboard. John woke up just in time, realised the approaching disaster, and yelled,

"Starboard." The other boat went about and then said,

"But I was on starboard."

"So you were," said John. I must add that John had already started a brilliant career as an advertising executive. We are still in touch.

Those are my stories of my dinghy sailing. I did some ocean racing, but my sea sickness meant that I neither enjoyed it or was of much use. Sea sickness tablets were available but in those days were fairly primitive and made one very sleepy. In dinghies I was regularly sick, and well known for being so, particularly on the day after a strong wind when the sea was still going up and down, but a dinghy race would only last a couple of hours and I would not become dehydrated. I could sail in racing yachts in Cowes weeks and did four or five in 'Grenade' a class 3 yacht belonging to Col Ken Wylie who for his retirement job after the Royal Artillery was the secretary of the graduate recruitment centre in Cambridge (Photo 21.4). At about that time I also did Cowes weeks in Daring and in Dragon racing yachts. Skippers wanting crews would advertise in the Island Sailing Club in Cowes, and from there we were recruited. The most incredible luck was when I crewed for Colin Ratsey of the famous sailmakers Ratsey and Lapthorne in his Dragon on the first day of that Cowes week. At the end of the race Colin asked me what I was doing for the rest of the week. I had nothing organised and was hoping that he would keep me as his crew. He then said that he was not racing again that week – would I like to borrow his boat.

In another Cowes week I joined an Australian surgeon who was sailing his ocean racing yacht with his attractive daughter. I must have impressed one of them as he offered to fly me out to Australia to navigate for him in the upcoming Sydney Hobart race. I had to admit to my sea sickness and tragically turned down what would have been my first visit to the country. Finally in my ocean racing very short career John Ogle not only owned his International 14 but also a racing yacht. He persuaded me that I could do a Fastnet race with him and his crew. The Fastnet race always started at the end of the Cowes week. We therefore met in Dover to sail the boat round to Cowes for the week beforehand. It blew a

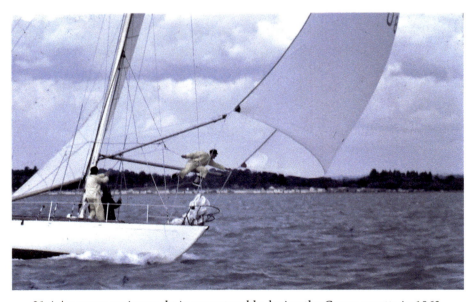

21.4 An ocean racing yacht in some trouble during the Cowes regatta in 1963.

force 9 headwind, and I was ill and severely dehydrated by the time we arrived in Cowes. I told John that very unfortunately it would not be possible for me to do the Fastnet, and could he please find somebody else. I was by this stage quite well recognised as a competent racing sailor and that week four other people asked me to join their Fastnet boat. I turned them all down, and what was so frustrating afterwards was that I could have done it with John as the wind did not go above a force 4 at any time during that year's race.

At Seaview I had regularly crewed Mike Jarman in Mermaids, and he asked me to crew in the Inter Services Gold Cup regatta. Our boat, which was one of the three from the Royal Air Force, was slightly unbalanced with Mike, a retired Air Commodore on the helm, an Air Vice Marshall as the middle man and an ex cadet, me, on the foredeck. It was an excellent two days, and we won the cup easily.

Finally before a gap of twenty five years in my sailing must come the Olympics. In 1969 Mike Jarman acquired a Tempest two-man keelboat. This was designed by Ian Proctor – who had designed my National 12 – and had been adopted for the 1972 Olympics. It was a fabulous boat to sail with a single trapeze for the crew, and my weight was just enough to be competitive. Mike asked me to crew him for a year leading up to the British trials which were to be held during Cowes week in 1970. I was about to go to Oxford at the time and as most of the regular sailing was to be at Grafham Water it was possible. We did consistently well and were always in the top two. And then came Cowes Week to select the boat for intensive training for the 1972 Olympics. For the first time we did less well and over the week only came fifth. The end of our Olympic dream. If we had been selected I cannot now see how I could have fitted in the work-up that would have been necessary. I would have had to postpone my medical degree a year, postpone my visit to the United States, and even postpone my marriage. So perhaps not too much of a disaster, although I would have postponed them all!

After the 1970 Cowes Week I gave up all sailing, and gave it up almost totally for 25 years. During those years I sailed once in South Africa, once at Seaview and once in Florida. The latter was interesting. We were over there as a family, and for some peculiar reason my two teenaged daughters enjoyed lying on a beach doing nothing. Within two days I was bored, and with the help of the local telephone directory contacted a plastic surgeon. I asked whether I could spend the next day with him. He said that he would normally have been delighted but had arranged with his son and wife that they would have the day sailing on his boat. And then came the unexpected invitation for the four of us to join them. So we all had a gentle sail and some excellent food and wine in the seas off Miami. What we did see in numbers and which particularly interested me were manatees, also known as sea cows. And it was another of those chance encounters. Although five thousand miles apart we had both been taught by Mr Hugh Brown, who had been my consultant in Newcastle and had taught him anatomy at a medical school in the States.

As I became busier and busier both at home and around the world, time for sailing became less and less likely. However in 1998 a new and extra consultant was appointed to Stoke Mandeville and my wife Vivian and I decided to purchase a property at which to spend the occasional weekend. We spent two weekends looking at properties starting at Salcombe in Devon and moving eastwards along the coast. When we arrived on the Isle of Wight, which Vivian had never visited, old and very pleasant memories flooded back to me and the decision was made. We bought a weekend residence which was part of Seagrove Manor and I then had to rejoin Sea View Yacht Club. Interestingly they insisted on a formal interview which I felt was somewhat unusual. One of the committee members and I spent most of the time talking about the club twenty five years earlier, and that was a time before the remainder of the committee had been members. We were accepted. As I said earlier in the chapter SVYC was unusual in that the Mermaid keelboats were owned by the club, and for insurance reasons anyone sailing them had to be assessed as to their competency and its level. Suitable helms were rated as "B", which was suitable for light weather sailing, or "A", which was for heavy weather. This assessment could be done at any time, but was most easily and enjoyably done during the Adult Week which was held in July every year. Vivian and I signed up. On day 1 I was a beginner, by day 5 I was an "A" helm and instructing. Sailing and cycling one does not forget. Vivian had not sailed previously and qualified as a "B" helm some four years later. Every year since then until Covid came along I have been instructing, and have also passed the RYA Keelboat instructor examination.

By this stage my National 12 had been sold, and I was somewhat long in the tooth for small racing dinghies. I therefore bought a very old Flying Fifteen. These are a two man keelboat which had been designed in 1947, again by Uffa Fox, and can be described as an old man's dinghy. Our first boat was extremely ancient and was turned into a funeral pyre after Vivian put her foot through the bottom. I replaced it with another, but Mermaid sailing really took over and I donated the second one to a youth charity on the Island.

Nearly all our sailing has been on the Island. There were a few unusual experiences. When I was examining in Abu Dhabi I hired a catamaran and took some of my fellow examiners for a pleasant sail. And when we were in Cuba the tour that we were on went for a cruise in a large twelve berth catamaran. Within ten minutes the helmsman handed me the wheel and I sailed it for the rest of the afternoon. The only two cats that I ever sailed. The other unusual boat in which I was given the tiller was a felucca on the River Nile at Aswan. An interestingly difficult boat to sail in a strongish wind as one had to pull really hard to keep the boat going straight.

And I may still be sailing and teaching until they put me in my coffin – and who knows about afterwards.

POWER BOATING

This is somewhat of a misnomer as most ocean going yachts have a motor aboard. However there are also boats whose only means of propulsion is an engine. These can be divided up into various types, and the commonest are either of solid construction or are Rigid Inflatable Boats (RIBs). The latter are smaller, faster, probably cheaper and easier to maintain. The soft sides are also very valuable when they are being used as rescue boats for coming alongside quays or solid boats. Requirements of the RYA yacht instructor certificate to be fully completed are that the instructor must also hold a basic powerboat certificate, a first aid certificate and a marine radio certificate. I therefore did the level 2 course and enjoyed it. There followed the advanced level 4 course which included night navigation by dead reckoning, and planning and doing a long sea voyage. By this time I had bought a somewhat unusual RIB that had an inboard diesel engine instead of the normal outboard petrol engine. We used this for the course and Gen Martin White (later Sir Martin) and I successfully passed it together. And with Covid the RIB now sits in a barn at home.

WINDSURFING

This is another form of sailing which is popular among the young. All four of us decided to try it, and in an almost calm day successfully did and passed a short course at Thorpe Park close to the M25 motorway. The next year we had a family holiday in Spain, and in the chalet was a windsurf boat. As a sailor and with my very basic certificate I took it to sea. Bad mistake – there was an offshore fairly strong breeze and I had not recognized that the boat had a light-weather rig. I very soon started capsizing and was becoming tired righting it. There was no paddle aboard, and I would not have known what to do with the sail if I had taken it down. Vivian could see that I was in trouble and asked a RIB to go to my aid. Very embarrassed I was towed back ashore, and that was definitely the end of my windsurfing career.

TWENTY-TWO

TRAINING AND OTHER SPORTS

Succeeding at, and also enjoying doing any sport requires a form or forms of training. This can be a specialist skill or skills, a specific fitness or general fitness. An example could be ice hockey which has been described as running a 100 metres for half an hour and where general fitness is extremely important. The specific fitness is skating – both forwards and backwards, and the specific skill is shooting the puck accurately at the net. I remember a friend at university who was a rugby player at a high level saying that one did not need to be fit to sail. On a windy day I took him sailing in a dinghy and showed him how to sit out to keep the boat upright. Because there is almost no movement required he had assumed that this would be easy, Ten minutes later his muscles had faded and he was pleading for mercy. He never complained again. General fitness is most often acquired by road running which can be very boring. Much more interesting was circuit training. This is done in a gym, and consists of doing a specific number of repeats in a variety of different exercises. For example one may start by doing five repeats of each exercise within a specific time, and when one reaches the target time the repeats rise to eight, and then to ten. This is often in competition with other people at the same time which makes it very much less boring.

Fitness training, no smoking and little alcohol as well as keeping my weight down were part of my life from schooldays. Without a doubt as I reach into my eighties they have helped me enormously. My blood pressure is still about 120/80 and my resting pulse under 50bpm, and I have never been overweight on the BMI scale. Perhaps surprisingly with the amount of sport that I have played I have needed no joint replacements, although one knee is minimally uncomfortable.

A brief mention of other sports. There are some sports which I have not even seen except perhaps on television. These include racquets, fives, boxing, lacrosse (despite a Cambridge girlfriend captaining the university ladies' team) and equine dressage, cross country and jumping. On only two occasions did I try horse riding and decided that being in control of a car or motorcycle was much simpler and more enjoyable. The thought of horse racing was not built into my brain although I can see the attraction of jump racing where skill and nerve are required. I do wonder whether flat racing would even exist without the betting. I have seen it at Ascot on many occasions when I have been on medical duty there, and have been very bored when watching. I have once seen polo. Certainly this was skilful and exciting, and has the tremendous advantage that age is not a major disadvantage. One friend, Tom Morrison, is still playing in his seventies. There are several other sports which can be played into older age which include sailing, golf, royal tennis, target shooting, croquet, bowls and snooker. I have tried golf and if I had had the time would have played more, but perhaps now a little too old to start. The royal tennis court at Cambridge was used more frequently as an extra badminton court, and it was only about ten years ago that a sailing friend, David Rowley, invited me for a game at the Hampton Court Palace Royal Tennis Court. It was clearly a game where the subtlety and skills that I had learned on the badminton court were relevant, and I actually beat my very experienced opponent in one game. Had a court been closer to the Island I would have continued, but it is a rare sport and courts are widely separated and one of our barns was a little too small to be converted.

At school Sgt Major West tried to introduce boxing. I was put into the ring with John Place in my form and we spent three minutes trying not to hit each other. I am a strong believer that any sport where one is trying to knock out one's opponent should be banned, and I am delighted that it is now recommended by the General Medical Council that no doctors should be involved. Also at school we did gymnastics at a very primitive level. I neither enjoyed it or was good at it. It does however run in the family through both of our daughters, one of whom broke both arms and still continued, and still continues through the grandchildren who are winning medals at National level. Another sport that I have not done is mountaineering. As a schoolboy I climbed trees – not without misgivings as I was definitely 90% wimp and only 10% brave. In later years I did some rock climbing but always without ropes, and was happier on sea cliffs where had I fallen it would have been into the sea. Probably my most difficult climb was Mt Isandlwana in Zululand, and having got to the top it was apparent why the Welsh army troops failed to escape in the Zulu wars. Not easy, and distinctly crumbly. My final major hill walking was in Sri Lanka in 2014. I did a relatively simple long walk with no falls or minor injuries, and the next day woke up with a very painful right knee. I needed a crutch, and it has not since recovered completely, and my tennis and cricket days are I think now over because of it. At one time in my life I nearly had to do rope climbing when I applied to join the Royal Navy Volunteer Reserves. As they were wanting a medical officer for the Royal Marines I would have had to do the Royal Marines green berry course. However a promotion within the NHS and a move of 180 miles from Birmingham precluded continuing my application.

Perhaps my weirdest near miss was Australian Rules Football. A match had been arranged between Oxford and Cambridge and Cambridge were one man short. I had never seen the game, but an Australian friend, David Sutherland, volunteered me. Luckily an Ozzie was found just in time, and it was only ten years later when I was taken to see a game in Melbourne that I realised that I would have been about six inches too short to have been able to play the game with any ability at all.

And finally two sports in which I would have been more involved had the opportunity occurred. Firstly motor sport. As soon as I started driving I wanted a sports car, and to race it if it had been possible. The one sprint race that I did with the Cambridge University Automobile Club at Snetterton finished half way up the track with my very broken MG TC. Clearly a sport that I could not afford. I became very involved with motor racing much later in my life as a qualified doctor working at various tracks and hill climbs as a track doctor. I have done track days in my Caterham and have lapped Silverstone at 99mph, and also a track day in a Formula Junior single seater. I have also tried go-karting at Silverstone and at RAF Akrotiri. Great fun but I was too old to take it seriously.

The last sport that I tried was Judo. At Leeds, Roundhay Lake on which we sailed would freeze most winters, and with no sailing I had the opportunity to try judo. It was very different to any other sport that I had enjoyed at the time, but somewhere there was a natural ability and I was progressing well when the lake unfroze – and back to sailing. The one thing that I did learn from judo was how to fall, and it has been very useful since. Never put out a hand if you are falling – land on a forearm or shoulder and the chance of a fracture are much reduced.

As I said in the introduction sport has been a major part of my life. It has made and kept me fit, it has allowed me to travel to several countries, and although I have had fractures of a leg, an arm and a nose I would not have missed it for anything. My wife, daughters and grandchildren are all keen sportsmen.

A final thought. Success in sport is obvious when the fastest, the furthest or the strongest wins. Clearly many sports require an umpire or referee that are sufficiently trained. This is easier now with video recording which has enormously improved the accuracy of judgements in cricket, soccer, rugby etc. But one is left with a variety of sports where the performance is judged by a panel of judges. All of these sports require physical ability but also have an element of artistic input which is why judging is required. These sports include gymnastics, freestyle skiing, diving and figure skating. Bias and dishonesty are reduced when the top and bottom score are removed, but I still have doubts about the results in such sports. Should these remain as Olympic sports? Where does boxing come in? I am convinced that any sport or other occupation where brain damage is an aim should be totally banned.

Part Four
Religion, Politics and Race

RELIGION

In different times and in different places religion has evolved many times around the world. In almost all religions there is the involvement of an afterlife for which a person has to work in this life. Is the afterlife a necessity because we are not happy that we are going to die, or is it a necessity for the priesthood to have a bargaining point to make a congregation behave and to keep them – both spiritually and financially. To quote from Voltaire. "If God did not exist it would be necessary to invent Him". But whatever the origins of religions as well as giving comfort to many believers they have also without a doubt caused hardship, war and death to multitudes of people. So many of the last wars and conflicts have been caused by differences not only between religions but within religions, even when occurring within the same race. The Bosnian war was a classic example of this combination.

However as well as religion causing the deaths of many people both in wars and appalling occurrences such as the Inquisition and the conquering of nations it has often encouraged an increase in numbers of its members both in a belief of helping people, but also no doubt for political gain in democracies where every member has a vote.

Both improvements in nutrition, of medical advances as well as an increase in wealth in many countries have also caused a massive increase in the population of the world. But this has often been compounded by religions.

The opposite to breeding occurs most obviously in priests, monks and nuns of the Roman Catholic church – at least officially, and occasionally in other religions. The most interesting taboo that I have come across is (or was) among the Zulus where although more twins are born than in many countries, only one survives. This was presumably based on the fact that both twins were less likely to survive when nutrition was poor, as might a parent who was trying to feed them. There was a strong cultural enforcement to this in that men were taught that if both twins did survive then they would die.

Attitudes to contraception also vary around the world. It is still banned by the Roman Catholic church on religious grounds, although widely used by Catholics. The argument is that contraception interferes with the natural order of life and is defined as a sin against nature. This I have never understood as Catholics are permitted to use modern medicines or to have surgery and this appears not to be a sin against nature. The lack of logic in this has escaped the notice of successive Popes. The only forms of reducing pregnancy that are permissible are natural child planning based on the "infertile" period in the monthly cycle, and also child spacing. Many years ago I went to a lecture at the Royal Institution in London by Dr Malcolm Potts, an old friend from Cambridge days, who at the time of the lecture was the senior doctor in the Planned Parenthood Association. In the questions after an informative and excellent lecture a member of the audience asked Malcolm why he had not mentioned natural child planning.

"Ah yes," answered Malcolm.

"We have a name for people who use natural planning – we call them parents."

When my wife and I were working in Lesotho, which is predominantly Catholic, child spacing occurred. By breast feeding a newborn baby for up to two years this markedly reduced the chance of another pregnancy. This was and is allowed by the church.

As the greatest danger that I foresee for the future of mankind is the increase in human population. For a previous Pope to go around and say, "Breed my children," is to me the making of a complete and future disaster, compounding global warming, destruction of forests and of natural habitats, and of increasing hunger.

A further problem has been both attitudes and the legal situation of countries and of religions to abortion. I personally believe that the term abortion should only be used for natural abortions which are happening all the time, and the word termination when it is done by humans to finish a pregnancy. Terminations are always unfortunate and often the cause of mental problems for the mother. I believe that they should be divided up into three groups, and the law should consider them differently. In the first group are terminations to save the life of the mother, and I am convinced that all religions and countries should allow these. The second group are terminations when there is known to be an abnormality of the foetus, for instance Down's syndrome. A child who is either severely mentally or physically abnormal puts enormous stress on the parents, other members of the family, and on the social and health services of a country. There is a strong case for termination in this situation. The third group where the termination is for convenience is much more difficult to justify, and especially where birth control methods, where they are allowed, are readily available. I am pleased that I was not a gynaecologist and had to make decisions whether to terminate or not.

Meslier (requoted by Diderot) wrote "And with the guts of the last priest let's strangle the neck of the last King." Which I have also seen quoted with the King replaced by politician. Would that it was true. Religion though is only partly to blame for the increase in the world population. When countries become rich, nutrition improves, disease becomes less and medicine advances. In Victorian times in England these all occurred together and a family would often have eight, ten or even more children. During Victoria's reign the population in the United Kingdom increased by 61% from 25.5M to 41M. When I was working in Africa many years ago, I would debate within myself whether I was doing the correct thing keeping people and particularly babies alive. The number of children that women had was determined by both culture and medicine. Modern medicine has revolutionised the survival rate of the populations, but cultural changes take much longer. I remember asking a pregnant lady whether she wanted any more children, and the answer was on two levels. Firstly that her husband expected her to have more children, and if she did not get pregnant when he returned from working in the mines, he would suspect infidelity. A completely illogical conclusion as had she been 'playing away', she would more likely have become pregnant. The second reason that she gave me was that her parents, basing it on their own experience, had told her that more than half her babies would die. And although this was indeed based on accurate history, the memory had not kept up with the changing facts of modern nutrition and medicine.

Another cultural problem that I have come across in both China and in India is the requirement to have a male offspring. In China the family line is through the male. One very good and extremely intelligent Chinese friend had two sons. I once asked him what would have happened if they had been daughters. He said that would not have been a problem, and then a couple of minutes later,

"But my parents would have been very upset." Which I do believe contradicted his view that it would not have been a problem to him as well as to his parents.

And the failure of the Chinese one child policy which one would imagine could have worked in China if anywhere in the world failed, because of the number of female foetuses that were aborted or female babies that were allowed to die. During the life of this policy there were 120 males for every 100 females born that survived, leaving a major problem for future marriages.

In India, a male offspring is still frequently considered essential as their future wife moves into the husband's family home to look after his parents. And in many countries and communities around the world several offspring are an advantage to look after the crops and livestock.

The population of the world, and in particular in developing countries, is increasing rapidly. Feeding this population is becoming increasingly difficult and is necessitating cutting down and clearing native vegetation, manufacturing and using fertilisers which also damage local natural history as well as needing large amounts of energy for their manufacture, and pesticides and herbicides which it is now being realised do enormous damage to pollination amongst other problems. Water supply is also becoming more and more difficult, both for drinking and for agriculture. It has been said that the next war will be over water availability, and the problems occurring now between Egypt, Sudan and Ethiopia may lead to a major war.

And more immediate is the problem of global warming which exacerbates many of the problems mentioned.

Is there an answer? With changes to religions and to local cultures it would be possible, but I am doubtful that it will be in time without a pandemic even more severe than the present one, or a total disaster such as a meteorite strike. The only hope in the future is education. In India the only state with a stable population is Kerala, and they have the highest rate of education of any state in India, and particularly of their women. So should foreign and charity aid from the rich countries only be used for education? There is an excellent case if we want to save the human race.

PERSONAL RELIGION AND POLITICS

I know nothing of my father's religion, the fact that he was a strong Freemason meant that he must have been a believer of some form. My mother had been a member of the Methodist Church as a young woman, and had even signed the pledge that she would refrain from alcohol for all her life. This turned out to be not quite true, but was not far off the truth – perhaps because she could not afford it. I do know that in my time as a child she never went to a church except for a wedding, and presumably a funeral. My own religious background started by being baptised. I had at least two Godmothers, one of whom had been the bridesmaid at my parents' wedding. Certainly there was one Godfather whose family owned the local building company in Buckhurst Hill for whom I worked during some school and university holidays. During the war I have no memory of anything religious in any form although services would have been held in the various Royal Air Force stations where my father was stationed.

When my mother and I returned to Buckhurst Hill after the war, at the age of eight, I joined the local cubs at All Saints Church, Woodford Wells. In 1946 the Scout movement was for boys only, although the leaders could be female. It was then a strongly rigid religious organisation incorporating all the churches. I would therefore have taken the Cub promise to do my duty to God, and would have been expected to attend church services. At about the same time, I joined the choir of All Saints, Woodford Wells. Being a choirboy required attendance at practice one evening a week, and going to church twice every Sunday to sing at Matins and Evensong. I also attended Sunday school every week during this time.

All Saints Church, Woodford Wells was relatively modern, having being built in 1874, with additions in 1876 and 1885. It was mock Gothic in design, and had a completely open southside across some of the beautiful grassland of Epping Forest. The vicar when I joined it was the Reverend Lemon, and it was on the conservative side of the Church of England, although not Anglo-Catholic. The choir master and organist was Mr Andrews, who had been the choirmaster for several years, was an excellent musician although interestingly he had the most appalling voice when he was singing and trying to demonstrate to us how we were meant to be singing. In those days the choirboys were all trebles, there were no girls. The Alto was a counter tenor and there were tenors and basses, again all men. As I became older, at Bancroft's School, regular church services were also held with a short service every morning and that was six days a week. There was a chapel at school, but my main connection with the chapel was pumping the organ for the school organist Roger Fisher. He later became the organist at Chester Cathedral. The school itself was non-denominational, but in fact was probably 80 to 90% Church of England with a very few Roman Catholics and, in my year, one Jewish boy. We had regular religious instruction from the school chaplain, although I cannot remember anyone doing divinity as an 'O' level exam.

At the age of 13 I virtually automatically became confirmed by the Bishop of Chelmsford in St Barnabas's Church, South Woodford. At the age of 14 I became a server in All Saint's Church, Woodford Wells, and was also on occasions the crucifer. The most outstanding occasion because of this latter post was when I met and spoke to our local member of Parliament – Mr Winston Churchill. There are some memories which one does not forget.

In the succeeding years I remained strictly Church of England, but in 1955 or 1956, very unfortunately the Rev Lemon committed suicide. Apparently this happened because his wife wanted a divorce. He did not believe in divorce, and to give her her freedom took an overdose in an hotel room. His place was taken at all Saints Church by the Rev Goodwin-Hudson who had been a missionary in South America. He was very much on the evangelical side of the church. His preaching was renowned, and he actually filled the church, often with younger people. However several of us were unhappy with the happy-clappy background of the vicar and his new services and we moved to St Barnabas's Church in South Woodford, which was very definitely Anglo-Catholic.

At this stage I was considering becoming a minister in the Church of England. My commitment however was not so total that I wished to go straight to a theological college, and I therefore went to the University of Leeds to read engineering. At Leeds, six of the seven of us in the digs were all strong believers. Both Roger Dunn and Neil Stevenson were Strict Methodists. Two of us were strong Church of England and the others were believers but not avid churchgoers. I first went to Saint Peter's Church, Bramley in the part of Leeds in which were my digs. I continued as a regular church goer and remained involved in the Scout movement and also its regular churchgoing.

However in my third year at university I accepted a place in Devonshire Hall of Residence. Devonshire Hall was built on the architectural form of an Oxbridge college. The rooms were based on the staircase formation, and this frequently meant that late in the evenings we would meet in somebody's rooms on our staircase for discussions. One of the other men on my staircase had communist leanings and certainly believed in true communism as the way forward. We would argue religion on a regular basis, and it became clear to me that my belief in various parts of the Bible, and in particular the Trinity, the Virgin Birth and the Resurrection were not sustainable with my scientific training and thoughts. I found it very difficult at the time, but eventually left the Church of England.

When I went to the University of Cambridge, religion both in college and in the University had a strong basis. Many of my friends were strongly religious, especially Leo Pyle, another engineer with me and a very strong Roman Catholic. His argument was that a religious belief was independent of his training as a scientist. Leo was Secretary of the Newman Foundation for Roman Catholics at all Universities. He wrote a book which was published at the same time as his PhD thesis about birth control in the Catholic Church, and for which he was nearly excommunicated. But also in Cambridge I was introduced to the Cambridge Humanist Society. This was a remarkable group of people with the most outstanding discussions. Among the group were Francis Crick, the Nobel prize winner for his discovery of DNA, and E M Forster the famous author. Joining in these discussions made it much clearer to me that I was no longer a Christian, but I remained as an agnostic. The Humanist movement has members varying from practising church goers to total atheists. I could not see there was any belief possible in the Trinity or the virgin birth, but equally I could not see any evidence that there was no supreme being looking after or involved with us in our time on earth. I had (and have) no belief in an afterlife, no belief in ghosts or any of the other accoutrements of religion, which to me were the strange beliefs of the Church of England and of the other various forms of Christianity, and in fact of several other religions.

I have remained in my belief in the humanist movement. At one stage in my time as a lecturer in London, one of my flatmates, Peter Burgess, became engaged to a Roman Catholic girl, and although he was a strong member of the Church of England felt that he ought to convert to Roman Catholicism. My belief in the Church of England had as I have said already gone, but my belief in the Roman Catholic Church was even less, and in particular I objected to the fact that anyone marrying into the Roman Catholic Church had to agree that their children would be brought up as Catholics. Peter went on to become a Catholic and I was the best man at their wedding which took place in the Roman Catholic Church of our Holy Redeemer and St Thomas More in Chelsea. At the lunch afterwards I was sitting next to the participating priest, Canon Alfonso de Zulueta, who was very well-known within and outside the Catholic Church at that time. We had the usual discussion about religion during the excellent, and well watered lunch, and halfway through he turned to me and said,

"I now see where Peter has been getting his arguments."

But the remarkable thing about Canon de Zulueta was that he invited me to talk to his congregation about humanism. In 1963 this was quite remarkable and a fascinating experience with the discussions that followed.

I am still an agnostic humanist, I still go to church for weddings, christenings, baptisms and funerals but still feel that the church has far too much influence not only in Britain, where it is clearly fading, but particularly in the rest of the world.

POLITICS

It is difficult to remember when politics became even a small part of my life. My mother was a staunch Conservative, and I assume that my father was probably the same. When we moved to live at home adjacent to Woodford Green it was a strongly conservative seat with of course Mr Winston Churchill as our MP. When he retired from the House of Commons the seat was then combined with Epping and Mr Biggs Davison held the seat. The Young Conservatives were very active locally, and were an excellent way of meeting other young people. Unfortunately I could not afford to belong to them! I therefore probably missed out on several early friendships. I then went up to Leeds University, and night-time discussions, to some extent in my digs, but then very much more markedly in Devonshire Hall of Residence which tended to be about religion, politics and not surprisingly but less intellectually, the opposite sex. It was here that I had to decide what I really believed in. From my background, and my scholarships both to school and university I had, and still have, a complete and total belief that everybody should have the same opportunities in life. It was obvious to me, particularly from my friends in the Hall of Residence that money also played a considerable part. With my scholarship to Bancroft's, I had to a large extent bypassed this condition. When I voted in the election, I voted Conservative. But I had very little other involvement in politics whilst at Leeds.

I then went to Cambridge where political discussion was more common than it had been in Leeds, and also, very often more intense. I certainly went to some conservative party meetings, and joined the University Conservative Association at that time.

I am not at all sure as to the reason, but when I became a lecturer in the

University of Surrey I became very much more involved in politics. I became a life member of the Conservative Association, and was also President of the University Conservative Club. In general in universities the Labour Party tends to be far more dominant than in other situations of work for young people. This was certainly the case at the University of Surrey. As the president of the University Conservative Club it was my duty to try to bring in speakers to address the club members. I had two major successes of which Enoch Powell was by far the greater. At that time he was Minister of Defence, but this was before the his famous, or perhaps infamous, Rivers of Blood speech. He came to the University to talk about defence, and met a very noisy and raucous audience the vast majority of whom were Labour supporters. He dealt quite brilliantly with the audience, and I always remember his technique. He said that as Minister of Defence now, anything that he did would not occur in fact for five or six years, and who knew then who would be the government. Again the defence changes that he was masterminding at that time had been put in motion by the previous Labour government. He then said, "Shall we talk about defence and leave the politics out of it."

There followed a fascinating hour of talk and questions to a receptive audience. The second person who came to talk to us was William Von Straubenzee, who at that time was involved in the Ministry of Education as an opposition spokesman, and particularly with universities.

When I went back to Cambridge in 1964, politics was no longer an important part of my life. I have always voted, though on occasions intentionally spoiling my paper when I disapproved of government policy, for instance about the Poll Tax.

I have since had one interesting conversation with Andrew Turner just after he was elected as the Tory MP for the Isle of Wight. He asked me if I had considered being elected to the County Council.

"An interesting thought Andrew – I might consider joining it as an Independent." For some reason he did not suggest it again.

RACE AND RACISM

Racial prejudice exists in almost everybody. Throughout one's life one reads both history and the everyday press, one has conversations and arguments, and one sees people of different races behaving differently, both personally and on television – and prejudice develops. It is always assumed that this prejudice is against a race, but it may also favour a race. The other problem with this prejudice is sorting out whether it is race or religion that is causing one's views. I have had wide experience of living in and travelling in more than 100 countries and have spent over eight years of my life overseas. As a doctor one is welcomed by countries and by people almost everywhere, but I have been submitted to mild racial abuse, and probably jealousy as well, in parts of Africa and in Israel. It is not always race that can cause feelings both for and against a person. Try spending time in Australia, in America or even in parts of Europe in all of which nationality alone, and not race can cause prejudice. This is normally, but certainly not always, light-hearted.

The races of *Homo sapiens* have occurred by movement of humans around the world many millennia ago, and on settlement in an area, by development of characteristics which were more appropriate for the land where that settlement occurred. Archaeologists and DNA experts are now working out some of these migrations and interbreedings with, for example, our Neanderthal forebears. In more recent centuries there has been movement of different races, sometimes voluntarily by colonisation or migration, and sometimes in the case of war, captives and of slaves, involuntarily. Very often both of these have caused resentment, and where there are obvious racial or religious differences, these were sufficient for instance to cause the second World War. But in many countries, for instance the United States, there has been serious civil upset. In some countries including Britain, both by general acceptance and by law, these resentments have reduced. I can remember in the 1960s in London signs in the streets saying, 'Room to let. No Blacks or Irish.'

The study of migration would require a book on its own. Everyone knows that Britain used slave labour when it was needed in the West Indies to grow sugar commercially, and after the second World War we then brought in half a million African ex-slaves to do manual work in this country. When the Indian population was thrown out of Kenya and Uganda a large number were welcomed into Britain again to do the jobs for which there were no local recruits. Recently Germany in particular within Europe has employed Turkish and other migrants when labour was needed. Hong Kong is a similar situation with the controls that are now in place on a population who were guaranteed a different life. These are examples of racial migration, but movement within nations around the world where race or religion is not a factor is occurring and increasing. For instance 4% of the population of

Greater London are French nationals and the many Russian oligarchs are now in the news. Illegal migration from Africa and from the Middle East into Europe, both to escape violence and for economic reasons is currently a major problem, and proving very difficult to control. As a by-product it is without doubt increasing racial resentment and unfortunately not only against the illegal migrants but other migrants who are here already completely legally.

Trying to analyse racial differences is extremely difficult. People are not born equal even within one race, but analysis between races is even more difficult. There may be differences in height, build, skin colour, facial characteristics, athletic ability, eyesight and perhaps even intelligence. Many or perhaps all of these are controlled by our DNA and are more consistent within a single race, but there are still major individual differences. Also there can be differences in childhood nutrition, in education, in physical ability and in attitude. Some of these can be easily measured, but the measurement for instance of intelligence is known to be very difficult and can be based on education which varies within countries and races. And what does one mean by intelligence anyway?

My favourite true story about attitude to life comes from Malawi. A new form of mealies (corn) had been produced which gave double the crop. It was given to some farmers to evaluate. One farmer and his family were just surviving by working very hard on the area of land that he owned. Two years later he was revisited to see what he was doing with the extra money that he was making. They discovered that in the second year he had planted only half his land, and was very happily sitting in his chair for many more hours each day. I cannot sometimes help feeling very envious of his attitude to life and sometimes wish that I also had it.

On a personal basis what I think is most important is that although people of the same race or of a different race may be different ,everybody should have an equal opportunity to compete in every way for work or entertainment or sport, and success should never be based on race, nationality, creed or sex.

The "Black Lives Matter" movement that is circulating around the world in 2020 offends me. If I started a movement saying "White Lives Matter" I would probably be arrested. Or if other people started movements saying Jewish, or Chinese, or Indian lives matter then these would be offensive to many people somewhere.

"All lives matter" I would totally support.

SUMMARY

As one finishes this volume of my memoirs one does wonder what was the value of the time that I have spent researching and writing it. Hopefully it may make some money for the medical research trust that I set up thirty years ago, and certainly it has given me something to do during the lockdowns caused by Covid – 19. It has also proved interesting and brought back many memories, mostly happy, of the past eighty years.

I realise how important was that first scholarship to Bancroft's School. From the day that the new bugs, as we were called, entered the school it was made clear that a major purpose of our education was for us to be going on to university to continue with our education, and in the 1950s only 2% of the population did so. The school was successful as eight of the sixty of my admission year became university lecturers, and three of us were admitted to the Order of the British Empire. The scholarships that followed were obviously important but perhaps to a lesser extent. However the income from them was crucial to me as the family had almost no money. How it happened is less obvious. I inherited three major advantages, I was intelligent, with an IQ measured at Cambridge of 164. I had a near photographic memory which made passing exams much simpler, and thirdly I have always believed in having a go at doing something different or unusual, whenever the chance was offered to me.

From my start with an absent father and a mother, who although extremely intelligent was almost uneducated, but who continually pushed me throughout my early life the background was somewhere there. And my childhood TB which lasted about two years causing me to miss two years of primary schooling must also have been a factor and could have been disastrous.

I am still astounded that I have finished up with seven degrees from three universities, and a string of letters after my name as well as professor before it. I have worked or taught in 45 countries and operated in 25 of them. And I have a wife, also a doctor, with whom I celebrated our golden wedding this year in our 14th century manor house in which we live surrounded by our own nature reserve. We have two daughters both succeeding in their lives, and they have two children each.

And I am still teaching.

And more and more I believe in the old adage.

Sudden death is nature's way of telling one to slow down.

AFTERTHOUGHTS

When Covid came along two years ago my teaching, travelling and normal life with local charities and friends went on to hold. What was I going to do in my spare time? Over several years people have suggested that I should write my memoirs. As I had travelled and worked around the world to work and to teach in forty-five countries this might be of interest. Also the history of my experiences and my work in wars and disasters worldwide would be recorded. My thoughts on how the health services and the teaching had altered during the 50 years since my medical qualification could also be involved.

I could see that my memoirs might be of interest to my family of future generations, and of course there is always the vanity involved in such an undertaking.

I am going to die within a few years. I do not believe in any religion and therefore will not expect the afterlife that so many religions promise. There is always the question as to how long one achievements, failures and aspirations last after one's death. There are many people who are well known or even famous during their lifetime. There are very few people whose reputation was such when they were alive that they are still recognised fifty, a hundred or even more years after their death. Clearly in the United Kingdom the kings and queens are such people. There are also famous politicians such as Sir Winston Churchill whose fame will last for many centuries after his death. However if one asked a normal person now to name other prime ministers over the past 100 years, I wonder how many would manage more than perhaps five or six. Going back more than a hundred years, I doubt if many, or if any, could be named. I'm sure this is also true with a few exceptions in the United States and in many other countries.

Another group of people who are remembered for many years are generals and other war leaders such as Bonaparte, Nelson and several Roman and Greek military leaders. A further group of people who are also remembered are philosophers, writers and poets. The reason that these are remembered is that their thoughts and actions at the time were written down.

And then there are people involved in wars and disasters such as Hitler and other people who have caused multiple deaths and destruction. I do know that my name would be remembered for hundreds of years if I had assassinated the late Queen Elizabeth when I was in close contact with her during my duties with the Royal Protection Group.

A more normal thought in the background when I started writing my autobiography was how would I be remembered? Clearly my work, and my operations on many thousands of people over the years would be remembered by those patients, and perhaps their families - hopefully because they worked and were successful, and made a difference to their lives. But when the patients die their memories would be lost. In the field of surgery there have been people who are now remembered because they have either described a condition or an operation. Examples of these are people such as Addison and Dupuytren. But for some unknown reason there has been for many years a movement to remove personal names from such diseases, and particularly anatomical structures, and to rename them with ordinary words. I have invented only one operation and although this is used, it has not got my name attached to it. I have been involved in writing nearly one hundred scientific papers, and also five book chapters , and now these volumes of my memoirs. Who knows how long my research will remain read as its significance was regrettably not as important as the discovery of penicillin or other world shattering work. Will it even remain available in book form or on the Internet? One advantage of writing a book in the United Kingdom is that a copy is held in the British Library.

There are other ways of being remembered, again in the United Kingdom an entry into works of reference such as *'Who's Who'* and *'People of Today'*. I was entered in the latter, but this has now gone onto the web and is no longer an annual printed volume. What has really changed is the introduction of Wikipedia. When writing these memoirs and trying to find information about people who have taught me, or with whom I have worked it was very much easier if there was a Wikipedia entry. My daughter Tasha is entering me at present and has told me that it is a difficult and time consuming effort.

It has been interesting that within my own family, because my parents split and divorced when I was very young my efforts to find information about my father's side has been remarkably unsuccessful. Through the efforts of a cousin, Marilyn, my mother's background has been traceable for nearly 3 centuries. My wife's family with the, probably unique, name of Onians has however been documented for many centuries.

And chance can also be involved in history. The Manor in which we now live has a complete list of owners going back to the Earl of Wessex in 1065, who became King Harold before he was killed at the Battle of Hastings. He precedes three other kings who have owned the Manor over the centuries. We are now on that list, which is an important part of local history. At least our names will be remembered, but very little else about my wife and myself. Around the house I have created the Roberts Nature Reserve which has been left in my will to a charity, and one of the conditions of the gift is that the name should be maintained. We are to be buried there and our tombstones will hopefully remain for some time.

A question that has to be answered is does it matter if our lives are recorded and remembered? Again vanity is a major factor, but it would have been interesting for me to have discovered much more about my own family history, and hopefully this will also be relevant to my descendants.

The final question is whether the human race will continue to exist at all, and is there therefore any relevance to having one's name and achievements in the historical record. Clearly at present with the threat of nuclear use by Putin we may be close to extermination. The author Nevil Shute considered this many years ago in his book '*On The Beach*', where rabbits survived longer than humans! There are also other worries in the future for the survival of our race. Climate change is widely discussed, but at least can be controlled if the willingness is there. More difficult is the increase in the population of the world who need feeding, and this is also related to climate change. I can see the increasing numbers of people being more difficult to control, and even China has failed to a large degree in its efforts to do so.

And writers of science fiction have come out with other suggested ends of our present world. An interesting book about the world recovering a thousand years after a disaster caused by the total collapse of computing is the '*Second Sleep*' by Robert Harris.

Perhaps the only hope for the human race in the future is by settlement on the moon or other planets. If this happens, as is being discussed at present, then the human race might continue, but it will be in a very different form.

And after those depressing thoughts I look forward to my memoirs being published, and hopefully remaining available for many centuries.

REFERENCES

Period Piece
Raverat, Gwen
Published by Faber and Faber, 1974
ISBN 10: 0571067425

Plastic Surgery in Wars, Disasters and Civilian Life.
Roberts, Prof Anthony
To be published by Pen and Sword, 2023
ISBN-978 1 39906 848 2

The Jungle Book
Kipling, Rudyard
Published by Macmillan and Co, London, 1894

Doctor in the House
Richard Gordon
Published by Michael Joseph, 1952

The Treatment of Burns
Cason, JS
Chapman and Hall Publishers 1981
ISBN-10 0412159902

Do No Harm: Stories of Life, Death and Brain Surgery
Marsh, Henry
Published by Phoenix, 2014
ISBN 10: 178022592XISBN 13: 9781780225920

Tale of a Guinea Pig
Geoffrey Page DSO, DFC
Bantam Books 1981
ISBN 0-7207-1354-4

Burns and their Treatment
Muir, I.F.K., Barclay, T.L. and Settle, John A.D
Butterworth-Heinemann Publishers 1987
ISBN 10: 0407003339

INDEX

Abrahams Harold, Olympian 216
Accident Service, Oxford 68,70,72,111,128
　Acker Bilk Musician 8
Addenbrooke's Hospital, Cambridge
　46,101,104,202
Alexander Lord, MCC 196
All Saints Church, Woodford Wells 201,267
Allen Dr, Paediatrician 97
Allen Sister Chris 160
Allison Professor Philip, General Surgeon 74
Almond Dr John, Sailor and GP 245
Alpha Dinghy 240,245
Anderson Dr, GP Cambridge 72
Anglo-American Mining Company 49
Ann Arbor, Michigan USA 94,96
Arctic Lapland 150,235
Ashby, Sir Eric, Former Master Clare College 46
Asprey Miss Vicky 244,251
Association of Cambridge University
　Assistants (ACUA) 212
Association of Northern Universities Sailing
　Clubs 237
Atkins Professor, Tony and Meg 96,204
Aufdenblatten Eddie, Ski Instructor 225
Australia 100,176,179

Ayre's Rock, (Uluru) Australia 181
Badenoch Dr, (later Sir) John, Medicine 69
Bader, Group Captain Douglas 132
Badminton 199
Bahai Faith 113
Bailey Mr Bruce, Plastic Surgeon 179
Bailey-Jones Rev, Rowing coach 212
Bailie Miss Fiona, Plastic Surgeon 156
Bainbridge Peter, Sailor 241
Bancroft's School 7,39,139,187,196,200,205,2
　15,235,267,274
Banerjee Mrs Sonia, Plastic Surgeon 173
Bantu Affairs Department (BAD) 88
Baragwanath Hospital, South Africa 81,91
Barclay Mr Tom, Plastic Surgeon 171
Barker Dr Maggie,
　Paediatrician82,85,111,116
Barker Mr Anthony CBE, Surgeon
　77,81,85,111,121
Barley Mow Public House 7
Barnard, Professor Christiaan, Surgeon 46,90
　Barnes Dame Josephine, Gynaecologist
　79
Barton Dr Carol, Haematologist 70
Bateman Peter, Sailor 240

Batstone Mr John, Plastic Surgeon 136
Battersea College of Advanced Technology 26
Battersea, London 33
Battle Hospital, Reading 101,108
Beaverbrook Lord 168
Bedford, The Duke and Duchess of 231
Bemba Tribe 6
Bennett Antonia and Sir Reginald 245
Bennett Mr John, Plastic Surgeon 169
Bevan Professor Peter, General Surgeon 148
Biafra 53,60
Binns Rev Dusty 200,215
Birchenough, Arthur and Dorian 224,245
Birmingham Accident Hospital 138,141,149,153,203
Black Mr Michael, Plastic Surgeon 159,161,179
Blackwell, Sir Basil 76
Blount Sir Edward, SVYC 245
Bonham Miss Eve 214,245
Boreham Mr Peter, General Surgeon 138
Bosnia 263
Botswana 122
Bowen Mr John, Plastic Surgeon 169
Bradford Football Club Fire 183
Bradford Royal Infirmary 171
Bragg Sir William and Sir Lawrence 12
Braithwaite Mr Fenton, Plastic Surgeon 164
Bramley, Yorkshire 4,7
Braund Martin, Tennis Player 206
Breach Mr Nick, Plastic Surgeon 168
British Association of Plastic Surgeons 172
British Coke Research Association 3,11,14
British Council 113
British Journal of Surgery 133
British Schools Exploring Society 4,50,217
British Universities Sailing Association (BUSA) 237
Bronowski, Dr Jacob 15,25
Brooks Dr David, Sailor and Flatmate 2,250
Brown Mr Hugh DL, Plastic Surgeon 159,161,176,254
Brown Mr Robert, Orthopaedic Surgeon 174
Browning Mr Chips, Plastic Surgeon 175,179
Browse Professor Norman, General Surgeon 149
Bull, Dr Max, Selwyn College 45
Bull Dr Microbiologist 145
Bureau of State Security (BOSS) 81
Burgess Mr Peter, Flatmate 95,269
Burton Trophy 23,249,251
Caesarean Section 86,93,113
Calne, Professor Roy, Surgeon 46,106,149
Cambidge Sister
Cambridge 67
Cambridge Bulldogs 19
Cambridge Technical College 20
Cambridge University see Univ. of Cambridge
Cambridge University Cruising Club 16,239
Cambridge University Medical Society 43,46
Campbell Gavin, Broadcaster 217
Cape Town, South Africa 89
Caroe Miss Jane 243
Cason Mr Jack, Burn Surgeon 144,146
Cavendish Laboratory, Cambridge 19
Charles Johnson Memorial Hospital, Zululand 81,85,121
Cheltenham 15,138
Cheltenham General Hospital 138
Chemical Engineering 5,14,36,194
Chesterman Mr Patrick, Orthopaedic Surgeon 102,109
Church Missionary Society 82
Church of England 7
Church of Scotland 60
Churchill Hospital, Oxford 66,72,135137,142
Churchill Sir Winston, Politician 268,270
Clapham Common, London 30
Clare College, Cambridge 24,39,45,105
Clutterbuck, Dr Ernest, Chemical Engineer 27,36
Cobbett Mr John, Plastic Surgeon 168,179

INDEX

Cochrane Mr Tom, Plastic Surgeon 169
Cockcroft Chris, Sailor and Sir John 241
Cockin Mr John, Orthopaedic Surgeon 12,133
Colback Dr Raymond, Anaesthetist 162
Comline Dr, Physiologist 39
Computers 19,34
Congo 55,56
Conservative Association 29,70
Consultant 126,182
Cousins Mr Frank 11
Cowes, Isle of Wight 252
Cox Ann, Sailor 250
Crans Montana, Switzerland 76,230
Crawford Mr, Plastic Surgeon 165
Crick Dr Francis, Noble Laureate 269
Crockett Mr David, Plastic Surgeon 171
Crockford Mr David, Plastic Surgeon 159,163
Cutting Mr Chris, A & E 141
Dainton, Professor Baron Frederick 12
Dar es Salaam 210
Daring Class Racing Yacht 252
Darwin College, Cambridge 18
Das Professor Suman, Chemical Engineer 212
Davenport Mr Peter, Plastic Surgeon 169
Davidson, Professor John F, Chemical Engineer 18
Dawson Mr Dickie, Plastic Surgeon 142
Deane Mr Malcolm, Plastic Surgeon 156
Desai Mr Sanu, Plastic Surgeon 195
Devonshire Hall, University of Leeds 12,209,268,270
Diagnostic Peritoneal Lavage (DPL Test) 92
Dick Charlesworth and his City Gents 8
Dickson Dr Wilfrid GP, Clifton Hambden 72
Dickson Mr Bill MBE, Plastic Surgeon 172
Dirac Professor P A M, Physicist 19
Dixon, Dr, King's College, Cambridge 45
Doherty Dr Shelagh, Rheumatologist 94
Dragon Class Racing Yacht 252
Drake Mr David, Paediatric Surgeon 106

Draper's Worshipful Company of 7
Dreesman, Miss Helen 206
Dudley Road Hospital, Birmingham 148
Duffett George, Engineer 12
Duffy, Mr Peter, General Surgeon
Duncan Dr, Hospital Superintendent 124
Dunn Mr David, General Surgeon 106
Dunn Roger and Jacquie 6
Duthie Professor Robert, Orthopaedic Surgeon 73
East Reach Hospital, Taunton 141
Eastwood Mr Derek, Plastic Surgeon 174
Edwarda Mr Teddy, Plastic Surgeon 159,162
Ellis Mr Frank, General Surgeon 227
Ellis Professor Harold, General Surgeon 148
EMO machine (East Mitchell Oxford) 70,116
Enderby Dr Hale, Anaesthetist 170
Engineering Society University of Leeds 8
Epping Forest 215,218
Essex County Council 3
Evans Cmdr 13
Evans Dr Tom, Physician 197
Evans Mr David, Plastic Surgeon 136,156
Everett Miss Anne, Sailor 238
Everett Mr Bill, General Surgeon 104,106,149
Everett Dr Charles, Chemical Engineer 22
Fairgrieve Mr John, General Surgeon 138
Fastnet Race 252
Feenan Maj Paul and Clare 232,274
Fiddian Mr Dick, General Surgeon 135
Firefly Dinghy 235,250
Fishburn Mr and Mrs 4
Fitzwilliam College, Cambridge 18,41
Fleming Children's Hospital, Newcastle 159
Flowers Dr Colin (Dr Cauliflower), A & E 139
Flying Fifteen Racing Yacht 257
Flynn John, Architect/ Skiing 227
Ford Motor Company 10,56
Forster E M, Novelist 269
Fox Uffa, Sailor/ Designer 235,243,254
Francis Miss Clare, Sailor/Author 244

Franklin John and Sue Chemical Engineer 237
Freedman Mr Arnold, Chemical Engineer 27
Freeman-Atwood Jonathan, Musician 195
Freemasonry 266
French Equatorial Africa 50
Frith Colin, Athlete 216
Fulwood Hospital, Sheffield 165
Furness Roger, Hockey 223
Gaff Dr, Psychiatrist 130
Gardner Dr Martin, St Caths 21
Gartside Dr 6
General Medical Council 102,128,182,258
Gibson Professor Myles, Neurosurgeon 158
Gillham Dr Tony, Chemical Engineer 21
Gillies Sir Harold, Plastic Surgeon 136,183
Girton village and College, Cambridge 16
Gissane Professor William, A & E 143
Gooch Graham, Cricketer 197
Gordon, Richard pseudonym of Dr Gordon Ostlere 48
Gough Mr Malcolm, General Surgeon 67
Goulcher Dr Roy, Chemical Engineer 27,35
Grafham Water 243,253
Great Ormond Street Hospital, London 177
Groom David St Caths 223
Guinea Pig Club and Public House 168,170
Gunning Mr Alf, Surgeon 74
Hall-Smith Dr Patrick, Dermatologist 169
Hardy Dr Dick, Physiologist and Flatmate 29,41
Harrington Christine, Nurse 95
Harrison Dr David – later Sir David 18,25
Harrison Sister, Nurse 67
Hastings Sister, Mary 130
Hausmann Dr Walter, Physician 109
Hawks Club, Cambridge 135,221
Hayling Island Sailing Club 248
Haynes Mr Stephen, General Surgeon 138
Herbert Sir Alan (A. P.) 247
Herman Taylor Professor, General Surgeon 149
Herman-Taylor Richard, Sailor 149,241
Herndon Dr David, Burn Surgeon USA 146
Heron Brian, Sailor 250
Higham Professor Charles, Archaeologist 23,191
Hill Professor Dylis, Sociologist 8
Hobday Kit Sailor 240
Hockaday Dr Derek, Physician 69
Holt Jack, Boat Designer 235
Hook Mr Barry also see Stobart-Hook 210,244
Hornet Dinghy 240
Houldsworth School of Applied Science 5,6
Howes Dr David, Haematologist 111
Howes Dr Valerie GP 111
Hunter Dr John, Anaesthetist 168
ICI, Agricultural Division, Billingham 33,249
Imperial College, London 4,22,35
Indaba 117
International 14' Dinghy 235
Isandlwana, Zululand 85,210,259
Island Sailing Club, Cowes 252
Isle of Wight 203
Italian Airways 50
Itchenor Sailing Club
Jackson Mr Douglas, Burn Surgeon 142,146
James Miss Cherry, Sailor/ Dentist 237
Janzekovic Dr, Surgeon Czechoslovakia 145
Jarman Air Cmdre Mike, Sailor 253
Johannesburg, South Africa 89
John Radcliffe Hospital, Oxford 129,132
Johnston Davey, Ice Hockey 220
Johnston Prof I D A, General Surgeon 167
Kafue Nature Reserve 58
Kalahari Game Reserve 123
Kaufmann Mr Harvey, General Surgeon 152
Kaunda Kenneth, President Zambia 60
Keith Dr Colin, Sailor/GP 238
Keith Richard, Sailor 237
Kellaway Dr, St Catharine's College 45
Kennedy President John F 72
Kennington, Oxford 138

INDEX

Kent HRH The Duke of 271
Kent Dickie, Sportsman 193
Kilner Professor T Pomfret, Plastic Surgeon 136
King Edward VII Hospital, Durban 89
King Professor Maurice, Pathologist 53
King's College, Cambridge 15,24
King-Cox Stuart, Sailor 235
Kitzbuhel, Austria 228
Kleinert Dr Harold, Plastic Surgeon 179
Knight Roger, Cricketer 194
Kubelik Martin, Ice Hockey 222
Lammergeier – Bearded Vulture 113
Land Rover 54,115,116,118,158,168
Lawlor Mr Dennis, Plastic Surgeon 167
Lawson Professor H H (Buddy),Surgeon 51
Ledingham Professor John, Physician 74
Lee Dr Christine, Physician 69
Lee Dr Grant, Physician 84
Lee Mr, Surgeon 74
Leeds General Infirmary 158,173
Leeds University. See Univ. of Leeds
Leeds University Sailing Club 29,235,251
Leggatt xi
Leggett Dr D M A. Vice Chancellor, University of Surrey 30,40
Leribe, Lesotho 114
Lesotho 111,112,125
Lever John, Cricketer 196
Lishman Miss Hazel, Radiographer 204
London Corinthian Sailing Club 247
London Mr Peter, A & E 147
London University. See Univ. of London
London University Sailing Club 29
Longland Lt Col Tony, SVYC 245
Lords Cricket Ground 193,197
Louisville, Kentucky USA
Lowbury Dr Edwin, Microbiologist 144
Lusaka 50,51,54
Luton and Dunstable Hospital 134Maddock Dr Alfie, Chemist 23
Makerere University Medical School 54l

Mallick Dr Donald, Geologist 6
Marendellas 58
Marsh Mr Henry, Neurosurgeon 158
Maseru, Lesotho 112,117,120
Mattka Berbel 224
May Peter, Cricketer 193
Maylandsea Bay Sailing Club 212,235
McAdam Dr Elspeth, Paediatrician 69
McCandless Father, Ice Hockey 222
McCrae Mr, Engineer 6,9
McGregor Dr Alan GP 50,52
McGrouther Professor Gus, Plastic Surgeon 165
McIndoe Sir Archibald, Plastic Surgeon 136,164,168
McLeod-Carey Lt Col Mossy 244
Medical Research Council 145,148
Megaw Moira 40,202,206,210
Melbourne, Australia 166,167
Merlin Rocket Dinghy 245,250
Mermaid Racing Yacht 244,254
Merriweather Rev Dr Alfred, Botswana 121
Merron Mr Ken, Sailor 247
Message Dr Michael, St Catharine's College 41,45,47
Michigan University. see Univ. of Michigan
Middlesex Hospital, London 82
Military Surgical Society 158
Miller Professor, Anatomist 50,53
Milne Mr David, A & E 164
Milns David, Sailor and Flatmate 235
Milton Keynes Hospital, Bucks 246
Minton-Beddoes Anna 227
Mohan Mr David, Neurosurgeon 73
Molepolole Hospital, Botswana 121,122
Moles Mr Frank, Chemical Engineer 27
Morecambe Eric, Comedian 135
Morell Miss Tessa, Surgeon 74
Morris Stewart, Sailor and Olympian 248
Morrison Mr Wayne, Plastic Surgeon 180
Moshoeshoe Dr, Lesotho 112
Moss Stirling 220

Mott Dr R A 15
Moussa Mr Jag, Sudan 145
Muir Mr Ian, Plastic Surgeon 171
Murison Small 224,226
Musto Keith, Sailor/ Olympian 240
Namibia 123
Nankevill Dr, St Catharine's College 45
Nash Mr, General Surgeon 154
National 12' Dinghy 235,238
National Coal Board 3,15,18,25
National Health Service (NHS) 47,182
National Lifesaving Badge 209
Ndola 55
New York USA 95
Newcastle upon Tyne 148
Newcastle General Hospital 159,164
Newman Col A C, VC 190
Newnham College, Cambridge 105
Ngema Futhie, Nurse 88
Nixon Miss Roz, Sailor 238
Norfolk Kate 7
North Side Hall of Residence 30,31,35,191
North Thames Gas Board, Beckton Works 10
Norton Hall, Billingham 33
Nottingham 156
Nqutu, Zululand 81,92,121
Nuffield Orthopaedic Centre, Oxford 73,136
Nuffield, Sister 67
Nwozo Mr Jim, Plastic Surgeon 136
Nyanga Mountains, Rhodesia 125
O'Brien Mr Bernie, Plastic Surgeon 179
O'Neill Mr Trevor, Plastic Surgeon 177
Ogle Mr John, Sailor 247,252
Olympics 187,253
Onians (later Roberts) Dr Vivian, GP 76,109,114,120,124,133,135,155,161,204,230,254,274
Oon Dr Chung-Hau, Physician 202
Orr Mr N W M, Surgeon/Skiing 229
    Osler House, Oxford 63,213
Oxford and Cambridge Sailing Society 242
Oxford Region Burn Unit 182
Oxford University, see Univ. of Oxford

Oxford University Yacht Club 240
Oxtoby Dr Bob, Engineer 14
Page Geoffrey, Guinea Pig 170
Parks Jim, Cricketer 196
Parkinson's Disease 110
Pasma Dr Fritz, Lesotho 114,115
    Patterson Mr T J S, Plastic Surgeon 72,136,142
Pay Dr Andrew, Physician 109
Peet Mr Eric, Plastic Surgeon 136
Pennybacker Mr Joe, Neurosurgeon 72
Perz Dr Bob, Ice Hockey 239
Petrie Dr Chris, Chemical Engineer 23
Petty Cury, Cambridge 16,242
Pigott Mr Alan, Plastic Surgeon 159
Pinderfields General Hospital, Wakefield 171
Pittman Dr John, Chemical Engineer 22
Plastic Surgery 111,135
    Plastic Surgery in Wars, Disasters and Civilian Life xi,11 179,180,184
Plymouth 250
Potalski, Dr, Chemical Engineer 27
Potchefstroom, South Africa 90
Potter Mr John, Neurosurgeon 72,131
Potts Dr Malcolm, Anatomist 45,264
    Powell Mr Enoch, Politician 271
    President of Liberia 29
    Prest Mr Richard, SVYC 245
    Prince of Wales Cup 249
    Proctor Ian, Boat designer 238,253
Proud (Atkins) Meg 225
Pyle Professor Leo, Chemical Engineer 21,35,269
Queen Elizabeth Hospital, Birmingham 151
    Queen, Her Majesty 198
Queen Victoria Hospital, East Grinstead 144,18,177
Queen's Hospital, Birmingham 148
Queen's Scout Badge 209
Radcliffe Infirmary, Oxford 63,70
Ratsey Colin, Ratsey and Lapthorne Sailmakers 252

Rattray Taylor Gordon, Author 46
Reading University, see Univ. of Reading
Registrar (Reg) 126
Reid Miss Caroline, Plastic Surgeon 160
Reuben Drs Brian and Catherine 31
Rhodesia (now Zimbabwe) 58,123
Richard Lower, Sister 66
Richards Dr Max – President of Trinidad and Tobago 22
Riddle Mr Jimmy, Skiing 229
Roberts Dr Vivian, GP – see Onians
Roberts Ivy B M xi
Roberts Kenneth A N xi
Robins Mr Robert, Orthopaedic Surgeon 140
Robinson Margaret, Sister 164
Robson Professor Bob, Hockey/St Caths 223
Roehampton College of Education – later University 28
Roman Catholic Church 120,263
Rorke's Drift, Zululand 85,88,210
Rothwell-Jackson Mr Rex, General Surgeon 135
Roundhay Lake, Leeds 235
Rowley Mr David, Sailor and Tennis Player 258
Royal Air Force xi,144,196
Royal Air Force Gold Cup for Sailing 253
Royal Berkshire Hospital, Reading 102,109
Royal Burnham Yacht Club 211
Royal College of General Practitioners 112
Royal College of Obstetrics and Gynaecology 89
Royal College of Physicians 89,127
Royal College of Physicians and Surgeons of Glasgow 127
Royal College of Surgeons 42,65,88,106,113,127,134,142,148,168
Royal Dutch Shell Co. 25
Royal Enfield Motorcycle 7
Royal Harwich Yacht Club 240
Royal Marsden Hospital, London 169
Royal Oak Public House, 'Chapel' 134

Royal Protection Group 198
Royal Victoria Infirmary, Newcastle 158
Royal Yachting Association 236,254
Royds Mr and Mrs Jumbo and Tasha 232,274
Saad Mr Magdy Plastic Surgeon 156
Saas Fe, Switzerland 226
Sage Mr Greg, Botanist 29
Sailer Toni, Olympic Skier 228
Sailing 234
St Andrew's Hospital, Billericay 177
St Barnabas's Church, South Woodford 268
St Bartholomew's Hospital, London 105,135,164
St Catharine's College, Cambridge 16,30
St Edmund Hall, Oxford 75
St George's Hospital, London 89
St Helier Hospital, London
St James' University Hospital, Leeds
St John Ambulance
St Luke's Hospital, Bradford
St Vincent's Hospital, Melbourne
Samways Dr Diana, Physician/Skier 228
Sanders Dr Sandy, Guinea Pig and GP 170
Sangoma. Witch Doctor 59
Sani Pass, Lesotho 118
Scarborough 251
Schleinitz Dr Hank, Chemical Engineer 22,194,219
Schroeder Peter, Sailor 237
Scott Mr, Orthopaedic Surgeon 102
Scott Sir Gilbert, Architect 174
Scott Sir Peter, Sailor and Artist 242
Scouts 189,209,211,235
Sea View Yacht Club 30,210,214,243,254
Seagrove Manor, Isle of Wight 254
Self Graham, Sailor 241
Selly Oak Hospital, Birmingham 150
Senior House Officer (SHO) 126
Senior Registrar (SR) 126
Settle Dr John OBE, Burn Surgeon 171,174
Sevitt Dr Simon, Pathologist 144
Seymour Spencer Dr, Psychiatrist 130

Shackleton Keith, Sailor 248
Shakeshaft Dr John, Physicist 23
Sharp Prof David OBE, Plastic Surgeon 171,173
Sharpe Tom, Author 21
Sheldonian Theatre 101
Shell Research, Stanlow Refinery 11
Shotley Bridge Hospital, Co Durham 165,176
Siddique Dr General Surgeon 113
Silver Street, Cambridge 21
Silverstone Motor Racing Track 259
Simpson Professor Keith, Pathologist 69
Singh Dr, Anatomist 50,52
Ski Club of Great Britain (SCGB) 75,228
Skiing 76,118,224
Smith Dubbie 206
Smith Ian, Rhodesia 124
South Africa 80,116
South African Government 81,85,111,121
Southern Rhodesia 58
Soweto, Johannesburg 81,91,93
Spurway Professor Neil and Alison, Sailor 76,247
Squash 51,203
Squire Mr Mike, Orthopaedic Surgeon 102,104
Stallworthy Professor Sir John, Gynaecologist 80,93
Steavenson Dr Robin, Sailor 35,247,249
Stephenson David Chemist 6
Stephenson John, MCC 197
Stevenson Neil, Pharmacologist 6
Stillwell Mr John, Plastic Surgeon 176
Stobart-Hook Barry, Engineer., see Hook Barry
Stoke Mandeville Hospital, Aylesbury xi,129,142,178,182,195
Stork John, Sailor 13,235,247,251
Sudan 141
Surrey University, see Univ. of Surrey
Sutherland Dr David, Chemical Engineer 22,259

Sweeney Dr Brian, Engineer 44,706,204,205
Tailby, Professor S R, Chemical Engineer 27
Tanner Mr Brent, Plastic Surgeon 177
Tapp Dr Roger, Physiologist 39,45
Taylor Dr Graham, Electronic Engineer 29,235
Taylor Mr, Orthopaedic Surgeon 78,134
Teddy Mr Peter, Neurosurgeon 71,94,133,134
Telford Hospital, Shropshire 138
Tempest Racing Yacht 253
Teyteyaneng, Lesotho 113
Thames Estuary Yacht Club 239
Thomas, Dr W J, Chemical Engineer 27
Thompson John, Sailor 241
Thorne, Dr Chris, St Catharine's College 41,42,43
Thornton Research Centre, The 25
Thorogood Mr and Mrs Peter and Leonie 231
Thorpe Bay Yacht Club 240
Tomkins Sir Edward and Lady Gillian 231
Till Mr Tim, General Surgeon 65,66,68
Tower of the Winds, Oxford 63
Town Gas 11,15
Transkei, South Africa 122
Transport and General Workers Union 11
Treliske Hospital, Truro 139
Trenton, New Jersey USA 95
Trinity Hall, Cambridge 105
Truman Christine, Tennis Player 205
Truman Nell, Tennis Player 206
Tsetse Flies 58
Tuberculosis (TB) 52,78,85,187,274
Tubman Mr Winston 29
Tugela River, Zululand 88
Turner Andrew, MP, Politician 271
Tutu, Archbishop Desmond 48
Twickenham 191
Underwood Derek, Cricketer 196
University College Hospital, London 47
University of California 53
University of Cambridge 14,106,161,201

INDEX

University of Leeds 3,4,6,17,20,74,194
University of London 27,28
University of Manchester 22
University of Michigan 94,97
University of Nottingham 156
University of Oxford 47,94,202
University of Reading 22,96,241
University of Southampton 109
University of St Andrews 47
University of Surrey 26,29,40,201,226,271
University of Zambia 49,75,205
Vass Mr Alan, Gynaecologist 74
Vaurien Dinghy 237
Venereal Diseases 114
Verbier, Switzerland 227,232
Verlander Michael, Scout 211
Vernon James, Sailor and Flatmate 247
Victoria Falls 56,57
Volkswagen Camper Van 11
Walsh Mr Tim, General Surgeon 104,106
Wankie National Park, Rhodesia 56
Ward Dr Jonty 82,87
Warnborough Road 63,76
Warneford Psychiatric Hospital, Oxford 71,136
Warner Sir Edward, Chemical Engineer 3
Webster Mr, General Surgeon 65
Wellington Sister 66
Welsh Harp, London 237
West Sgt Major, School Gym Master 215
Weston John and Rita 31
Wexham Park Hospital, Slough 155,160
Whipp's Cross Hospital, Wanstead 64,177,216
Whiston Hospital, Liverpool 176
Whitchurch Cricket Club 195
Whitehouse, Mr, Chemist 9
Whiteley Roger, School 216
Williams Mr Arthur ,Gynaecologist 74,78
Williams Roy, Sailor 241
Wilson, Harold, Prime Minister 26,36,173
Winstone Mr Norman, General Surgeon 152
Witch Doctor, Sangoma 59

Withycombe, Mr J F R, Urologist 46,101,104,150
Wollner Dr Leo. Geriatrician 72,131
Woodford County High School 200
Woodford Green Primary School 187,193
Woodford Wells 193
Worcester College, Oxford 75
Wright Billy, Footballer 189
Wright Dr Gordon, Anatomist 39,105
Wright Mr Gym Master 208
Wright Tessa, Sailor 250
Wyche and Coppock, Boat builders 238
Wylie Col Ken, Sailor 252
Wynne-Williams Mr, Plastic Surgeon 156
Yates Miss Sarah, Nurse/ Skiing 90,227
Youth Hostel Association – Maldon Essex 44,246
Zambia 49,62,71,92,117
Zambia University, see Univ. of Zambia
Zambian Flying Doctor Service 55
Zermatt, Switzerland 224
Ziman, Dr, Physicist 15
Zimbabwean Ruins 58
Zulu(s) 81,87,263
Zulueta Canon Alfonso de, Priest 269
Zululand KwaZulu 49,83